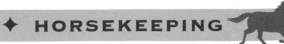

HORSEKEEPING SKILLS LIBRARY

Horse Health Care

A STEP-BY-STEP PHOTOGRAPHIC GUIDE TO MASTERING OVER 100 HORSEKEEPING SKILLS

CHERRY HILL
PHOTOGRAPHY BY RICHARD KLIMESH

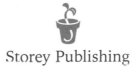

Storey Publishing

The mission of Storey Publishing is to serve our customers
by publishing practical information that encourages personal independence
in harmony with the environment.

Edited by Elizabeth McHale
Cover design by Eugenie Delany
Text design by Cynthia McFarland
Production by Therese G. Lenz and Allyson L. Hayes
Line drawings designed by Cherry Hill and drawn by Elayne Sears
Indexed by Susan Olason

The information in this book is true and complete to the best of our knowledge. All recommendations are made without guarantee on the part of the author or Storey Publishing. The author and publisher disclaim any liability in connection with the use of this information. For additional information, please contact Storey Publishing, 210 MASS MoCA Way, North Adams, MA 01247.

Storey books are available for special premium and promotional uses and for customized editions. For further information, please call 1-800-793-9396.

Printed in the United States by Vicks Lithograph and Printing

20 19 18 17 16 15 14 13 12

LIBRARY OF CONGRESS CATALOGING-IN-PUBLICATION DATA

Hill, Cherry, 1947–
    Horse health care : a step-by-step photographic guide to mastering over 100 horse-keeping skills / Cherry Hill : with photographs by Richard Klimesh.
            p.   cm. — (Horsekeeping skills)

        Includes bibliographical references and index.
        ISBN-13: 978-0-88266-955-9;
        ISBN-10: 0-88266-955-9 (pb : alk. paper)
        1. Horses—Health.   2. Horses.   3. Horses—Pictorial works.
    I. Title.   II. Series.
    SF285.3.H54   1997
    636. 1'083—hr dc20   96-34003
                                                               CIP

Contents

DEDICATION

To Klim-Click, my photo man

OTHER BOOKS BY CHERRY HILL

101 Arena Exercises

101 Horsemanship & Equitation Patterns

Horsekeeping on a Small Acreage

Becoming an Effective Rider

Your Pony, Your Horse

From the Center of the Ring

The Formative Years

Making Not Breaking

Maximum Hoof Power

Horse for Sale

Horse Handling & Grooming

Trailering Your Horse

Stablekeeping

Arena Pocket Guides

Horse Care for Kids

Acknowledgments

Special thanks to my husband and partner, Richard Klimesh, for his sense of humor and excellent help with the photographs.

Thanks to Sue DeGrazia for being a photo model. Also, thanks to my horses Zinger, Sassy, Zipper, Dickens, Blue, Aria, Seeker, and Drifter for their patience and cooperation as photo models.

I am grateful to the following for supplying products used in this book: **Ariat International,** for safe and comfortable boots; **BMB Animal Apparel,** for halters and blankets; **Les Vogt's Pro Equine,** for protective horse boots; **Miller's Harness Company,** for trailer boots; and **Cherry Mountain Forge,** for custom-forged blanket racks.

Preface

I really appreciate the fact that my photographer, Richard Klimesh, and my horses are so patient. They have gone way beyond the call of duty more than once during the photo shoots for this book. Sometimes we had to shoot certain sequences over due to sudden weather changes (wind, rain, snow) or lighting changes (whoops, the sun just popped out from behind the clouds) or freak occurrences (a cat strolls into the frame while I am bandaging). But it seemed like we could always depend on the horses to hang in there until Richard was satisfied and declared, "It's a wrap!"

Unfortunately, one of my horses made a rather painful contribution to this book. In the fall of 1995, we had a very early, heavy snow when the trees were still fully leafed. This caused many limbs and trees to come crashing down, leaving the ground littered with sharp branches. Aria, then just 24 months old, was out on one of the wooded creek pastures that day. She must have been in the wrong place at the wrong time because later she walked up to the barn with a major leg wound, which is illustrated in this book. So Aria became our model for bandaging a wound, following the progress of a wound, and giving an intramuscular injection. Thankfully, her leg healed well and she is currently in training.

The treatment of Aria's leg wound brings up an important point. I have designed this book to show you HOW to perform various skills. You will need to refer to other books for detailed explanations on behavior, training, facilities, nutrition, parasite control, immunization, and so on. See Recommended Reading for some suggestions.

Richard and I really enjoyed preparing this book. We hope it contributes to a healthy, happy relationship between you and your horse.

Safe Handling and Housing

EQUIPMENT FOR THE HANDLER

Although safety helmets are usually associated with riding, there are times when you are handling horses from the ground that it is a good idea to wear one. Protect your feet by wearing well-made, sturdy boots. Whenever possible wear gloves, especially when handling ropes. And always use safe horse-handling techniques.

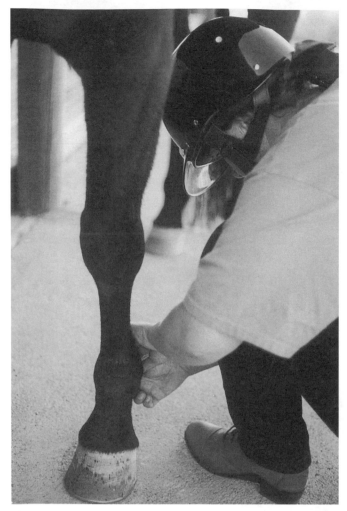

▲
SAFETY HELMET

If you are inexperienced or you are working with a young or green horse, it would be to your benefit to wear a protective helmet. When you are working on a horse's legs, the horse could accidentally hit you in the head when he stomps at a fly, or he could move suddenly and knock you into a wall or fence or onto the ground.

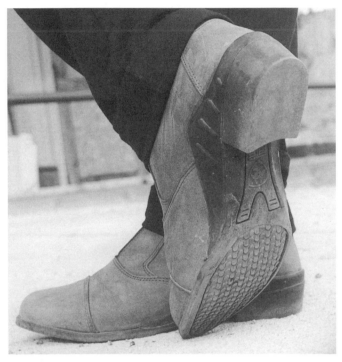

▲
STURDY BOOTS

Boots should have heels, good traction, and, if possible, an extra piece of leather sewn across the toe. This toe cap provides extra protection if a horse should step on your foot.

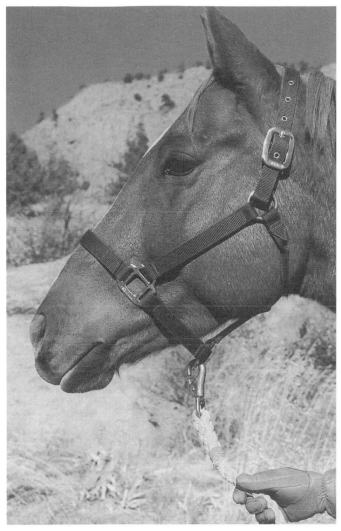

▲
STRONG EQUIPMENT AND LEATHER GLOVES

Always use strong, well-made, well-fitted equipment. Leather gloves will give you a better grip on ropes and protect your skin from the pain of a rope burn if the rope ever zings through your hand unexpectedly.

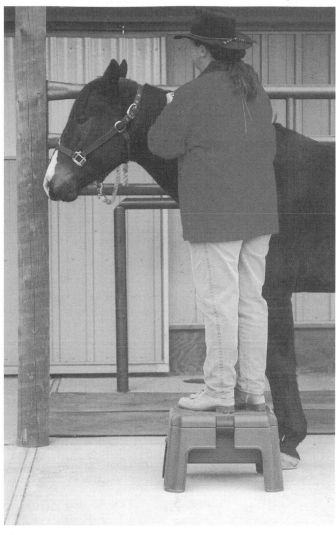

▲
STEP STOOL

When working on your horse's mane, if you need to get a bird's-eye view, use a steady step stool and place it next to the horse, not in front of him or underneath him. Also, if you have long hair, fasten it securely out of the way and wear a hat to further contain it.

HOLDING A HORSE FOR THE VETERINARIAN

When you are required to hold a horse for a veterinarian or you are acting as an assistant for a friend, there are certain principles you should keep in mind.

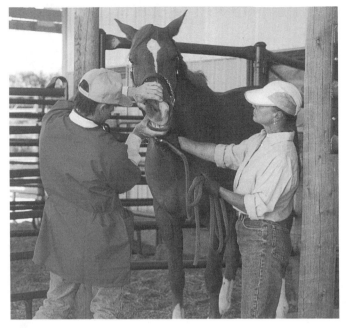

▲
HOLDING A HORSE

When the vet is working on the horse's head, hold the lead rope closer to the halter than normal so you can control the horse's head without the large sweeping motions that would be necessary if you held the horse on a long lead. Always pay attention to the horse's attitude and expression as the vet works; this will give you clues as to the likelihood of a sudden reaction. This handler would be in a safer situation if she were not backed up against the post. If the horse suddenly reared or moved away from the vet and the handler had to back up in a hurry, it could cause her to get pinned or hurt.

STAY ATTENTIVE ▶

Especially when the vet is working at the rear of the horse, stay attentive to your horse and keep him steady and straight. Here the horse is held alongside a strong pipe rail that keeps him from moving to the right.

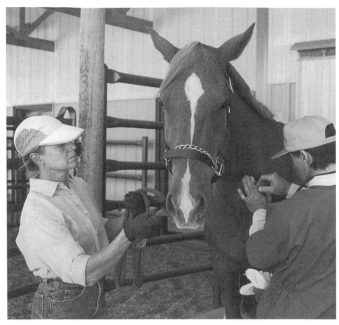

▲
A CHAIN OVER THE NOSE

If the horse needs a chain over the nose for complete cooperation and control, have the chain in place from the beginning of the session. If the vet is working on the near side to administer intravenous medication, for example, stand on the off side but with a clear view of the horse's expression and the vet's position.

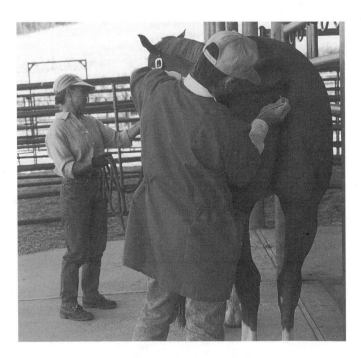

SAFELY HOUSING A HORSE

Whether your horse is housed in a stall or an outdoor pen, follow safe practices and provide safe eating and water areas.

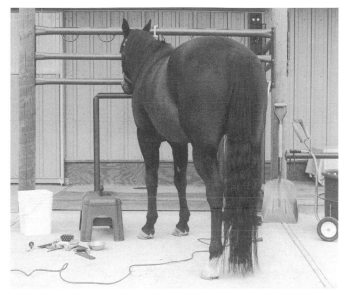

▲
AVOID CLUTTER

Follow safe practices at all times. Never leave a horse in a dangerously cluttered area like this. He could easily become hurt or damage your equipment.

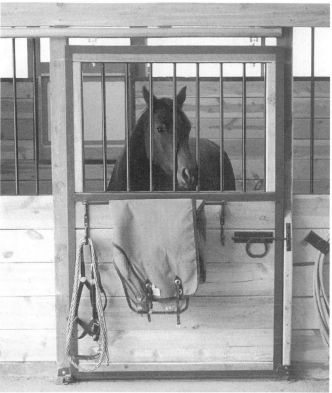

▲
THE STALL

Provide a safe, comfortable place for your horse to live. If your horse lives in a stall part of the time, be sure the stall has plenty of air and light; smooth, safe walls; and a safe feeder and waterer.

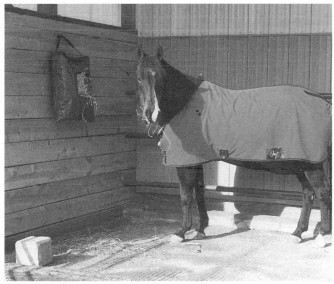

▲
OUTDOOR PEN

If your horse lives in an outdoor pen, provide him with a clean, safe eating area; shelter; and perhaps a sheet or blanket.

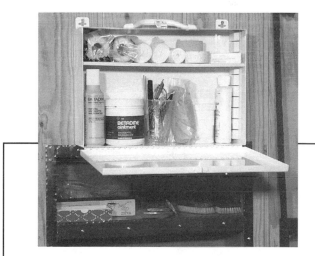

KNOW FIRST AID and have proper supplies and equipment on hand. Betadine, sterile gauze pads, conforming gauze roll, crepe bandage, scissors, latex gloves, thermometer, triple antibiotic ointment.

CLEANING A STALL

The cleaner you keep your horse's stall, the less chance he will have of reinfesting himself with parasites after being dewormed, the fresher the air will be in the barn, and the cleaner he and his blankets will stay.

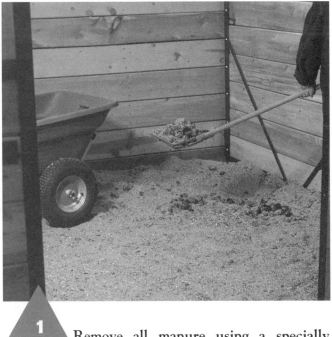

1 Remove all manure using a specially designed fork that has tines spaced close enough so that the manure does not fall through. These forks are available in plastic and metal. Certain metal-tined silage forks also work well.

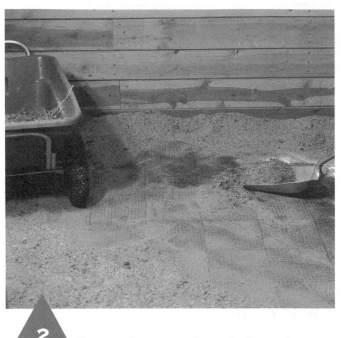

2 Locate the spots where the horse has urinated. The wet bedding should be removed using a scoop shovel. Aluminum or plastic shovels are lighter and easier to use than steel ones.

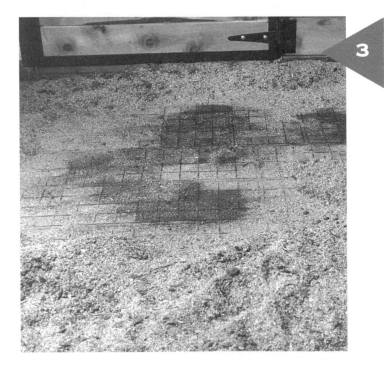

3 Pull all the bedding away from the wet spots so the base material can dry from exposure to air and sunlight.

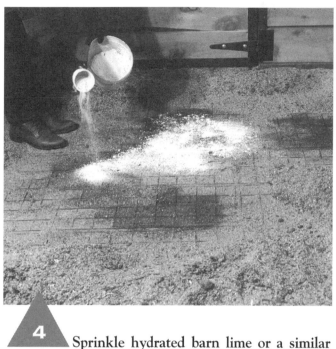

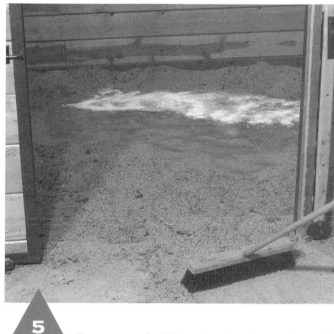

4 Sprinkle hydrated barn lime or a similar stall floor freshener on the wet spots. This not only neutralizes and decreases the smell of urine, but it also helps the floor dry faster.

5 Sweep any bedding that has been dragged out into the aisle back into the stall.

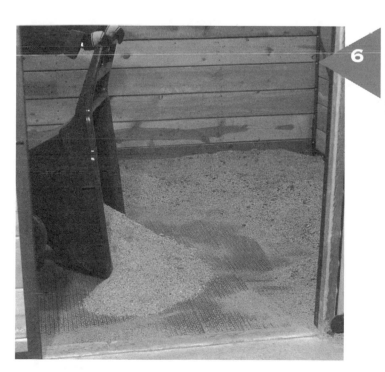

6 After the stall has dried, cover the area where the horse usually urinates with the clean leftover bedding. Add new bedding to the areas where the horse tends to lie down and eat.

Examining Your Horse

PLANNING A DAILY CHECK

Each day you should notice certain things about your horse so you can determine his or her state of health. Most of the following observations can be made at feeding time. (See also the upcoming skills: **Performing a Leg Check, Taking Vital Signs, Dental Check,** *and* **Hoof Check.***)*

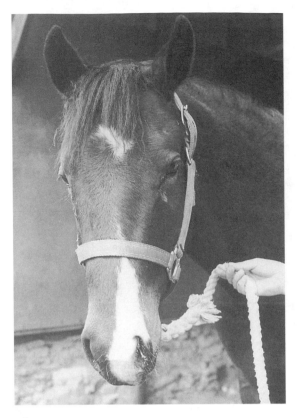

▲
EXPRESSION
Take a close look at your horse's expression and the condition of his eyes and nostrils. If you notice any discharge, as shown here, it might indicate your horse has a respiratory illness, such as influenza or rhinopneumonitis. Take your horse's vital signs, especially making note of his temperature, and then call your vet. (See **Vital Signs: Temperature, Pulse,** and **Respiration,** pp. 16–20.)

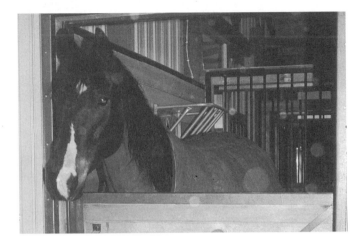

▲
APPETITE
As you approach your horse's stall or pen at feeding time, is he alert and eager to be fed? A good appetite is one of the most important signs of good health.

EXAMINE THE HORSE'S WATER PAIL OR TROUGH

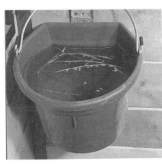

▲
A few hay stems or grains in the water are not cause for alarm because many horses flush out their mouths when they drink. Horses tend to drink about an hour or so after they have begun to eat the roughage portion of their rations.

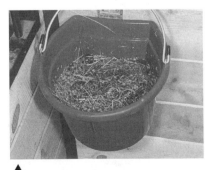

▲
If the water pail looks like this, your horse may be having difficulty eating and might be trying to soften the hay and grain before swallowing. This could indicate dental problems or a sore palate, tongue, or throat. Or the feed could have an off-taste.

MANURE CHECK

Keep an eye on your horse's manure because it indicates how his intestines are functioning, if he is drinking enough water, if he is suffering a digestive upset, if his food has been well chewed, and if he has worms.

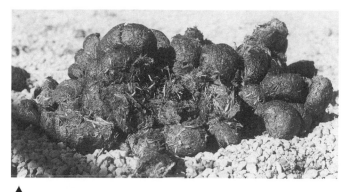

▲
NORMAL

Each horse will have his own "normal" feces. This is a fairly typical, normal, healthy horse manure pile: well-formed fecal balls with enough moisture so that the pile stays heaped. There is some coarse roughage that has passed through undigested. This is normal if you are feeding grass hay.

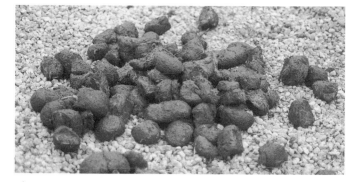

▲
DRY

This manure pile might be normal for some horses or it might indicate that this horse is not drinking enough water, since each fecal ball is quite separate and somewhat dry. This occurred during very cold weather when horses typically don't want to drink as much water as they should.

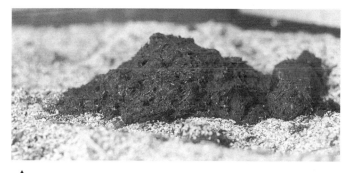

▲
LOOSE

This manure pile is loose with very little form to the fecal balls. This indicates that the feed passed through the horse rather quickly. This could be from a sudden change of feed from grass hay to rich alfalfa hay. Or it could be that the horse has eaten a lot of salt and drunk a lot of water. Or it could indicate a mechanical or bacterial irritation in the horse's gut. Some horses get a very loose stool when they are anxious or excited. And some mares have loose manure when they are in heat.

OFFER SUPPLEMENTS

Offer your horse a calcium-phosphorus (1:1) trace mineral salt block. A 40–50-pound block should be available to your horse at all times (one block should last one horse about a year). Keep a close eye on your horse's consumption of free-choice supplement blocks. If your horse is eating a particular block very rapidly, it usually means one of two things: (1) Your horse may be very deficient in salt or minerals and is craving them, or (2) the block that he has been offered also contains molasses and/or grain products, and he is eating it like "candy." This is the most likely reason a horse eats a block very fast. This can be dangerous because along with the sweet, tasty portion of the block that the horse is attracted to, he is also ingesting a large amount of salt that he doesn't need. Avoid the blocks that contain molasses and/or grain products.

CHECKING THE SKIN

One of the best ways to detect skin problems on your horse is to run your hands all over his body. Not only will this feel good to him, but also it will allow you to discover lumps and bumps that you can investigate further. If you are suspicious of external parasites such as ticks or lice, check the mane and tail carefully.

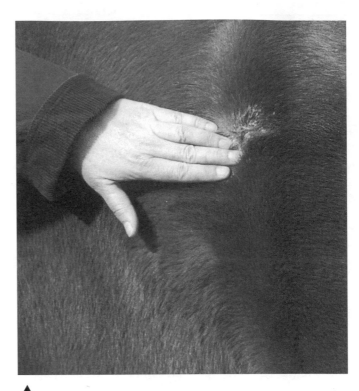

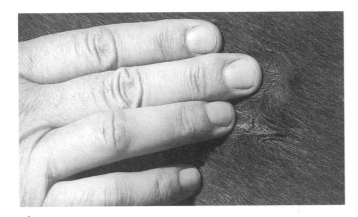

▲
SMALL WOUNDS
When you've located a trouble spot, investigate further by moving the surrounding hair out of the way. If you find dried blood or *serum* (the watery portion of the blood that sometimes oozes through the skin), the bump is probably a small wound that can be treated simply by washing with a good antiseptic soap and possibly applying a dab of antibacterial ointment.

▲
LOOK BENEATH THE WINTER COAT
This skin problem did not feel like a bump or a lump and the winter coat almost covered it completely. It will take some extra effort to check the skin when your horse has a thick winter coat.

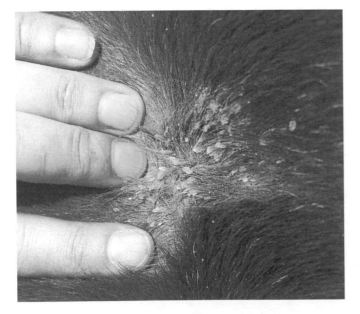

◀ DERMATITIS
A close-up shows that this is not an ordinary abrasion or small nick but a skin problem, often called *dermatitis*. In general terms, this means a skin irritation. If you see something like this, before you remove valuable clues to the cause by washing or clipping the area, have your veterinarian look at it.

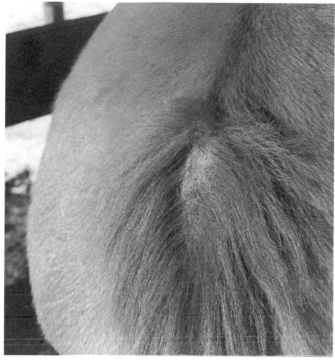

▲ CHECK THE MANE AND TAIL

If you see a bald patch like this on your horse's tail, it can indicate several causes of tail rubbing (from most likely to least likely):

✦ The horse's tail is dirty.
✦ The horse's tail had been shampooed and the shampoo was not rinsed out thoroughly.
✦ At one time the horse's tail was dirty or not rinsed thoroughly, and the horse developed the habit of tail rubbing and now just rubs out of habit.
✦ It is spring or fall shedding time, and the horse is rubbing many parts of his body to remove itchy hair.
✦ The horse has an infestation of lice or ticks.
✦ The horse's sheath or udder is dirty and since the horse can't reach these parts to scratch, he rubs the tail end.
✦ The horse has *Oxyuris equi* (pinworms) and the larvae (maggots) have crawled out of the anus and are causing an itch.

Good hygiene and a good deworming program usually prevent tail rubbing.

▲ SANITATION

The cleaner you keep your horse's buckets, feeders, and grooming tools, the less likely he will be to develop a skin problem or health problem. At least once a week, you should scrub out your horse's eating and drinking receptacles and wash the grooming tools you use on him. You can use regular soap or, if you suspect a problem, an antibacterial soap. Sunlight is also a great purifier, so let the clean items dry in strong sun. Let the bristle brushes rest on their sides as they dry so the wooden bases don't become waterlogged.

Various skin problems require different treatments, but follow these rules whenever you detect skin problems: Keep the horse's brushes, blankets, and tack separate from other horses'. Wash your hands between horses. If you use gloves, keep a separate pair for the horse with the skin problem.

PERFORMING A LEG CHECK

The condition of your horse's hooves and legs affects his comfort, soundness, and performance. A daily visual examination and careful palpation, particularly after strenuous work, can reveal swelling, heat, pain, or injury. Become familiar with the normal temperature, texture, and sensitivity of your *horse's legs so that you can detect when things are abnormal. (See the section on bathing and clipping in Horse Handling and Grooming to learn how to teach your horse to stand still while you are handling his legs.)*

ANATOMY OF THE HORSE'S LOWER LIMB

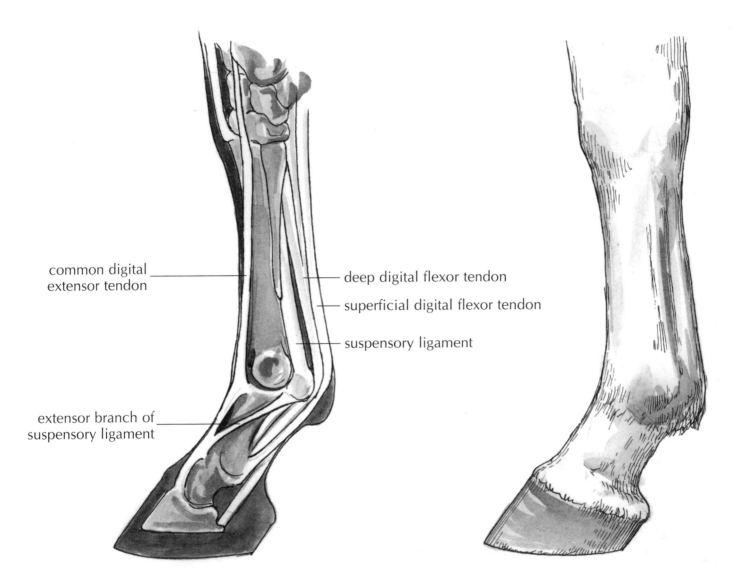

common digital extensor tendon

deep digital flexor tendon

superficial digital flexor tendon

suspensory ligament

extensor branch of suspensory ligament

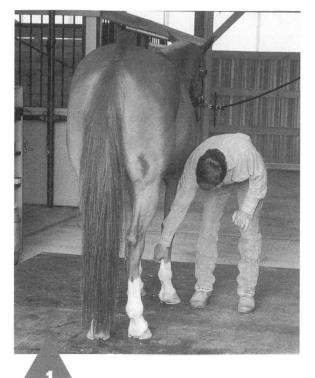

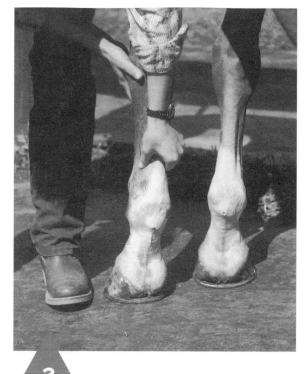

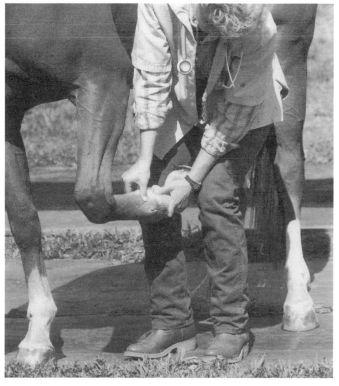

▲1 Establish what is normal for your horse's tendons and joints. With your horse standing comfortably on a level surface with his weight on all four feet, run your fingers down the flexor tendon area of his front legs to assess the temperature of leg tissues. Realize that if your hands are cold, his legs may feel warmer to you than if your hands are warm. Do the same for the hind legs.

▲2 While you are evaluating your horse's leg temperature this way, you are also getting an idea of what is the normal consistency and texture of your horse's lower limbs. This horse's left front leg normally carries more fluid around the joint and tendons due to an old injury. The right front leg does not carry excess fluid. It is "clean" and tight, which is commonly referred to as having "flat" bone.

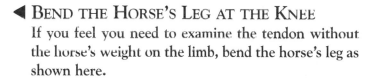

BEND THE HORSE'S LEG AT THE KNEE
If you feel you need to examine the tendon without the horse's weight on the limb, bend the horse's leg as shown here.

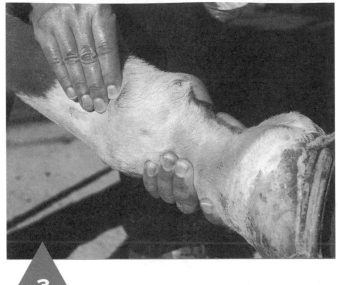

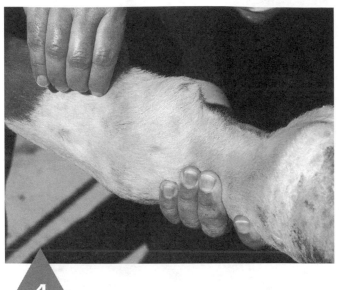

3 Feel the flexor tendon area for heat, thickness, or tenderness. Because you have previously checked your horse when you knew he was sound and comfortable, you will know what is normal for that horse and now you can compare the temperature of his leg, the amount of fluid in his limb, and his sensitivity to pressure.

4 Pick up the superficial flexor tendon with your fingers and work your way up and down the tendon to identify spots that might be more sensitive. Your horse will react quickly if you make contact with a sensitive area. Often a horse's tendons can be a bit sore after work, just like yours might be if you just ran a mile. In many cases, that would be normal. But persistent or worsening tendon soreness can signal poor conditioning, problems with shoeing or footing, and the possibility of an inflammation of the flexor tendon called *bowed tendon*, which your veterinarian should treat.

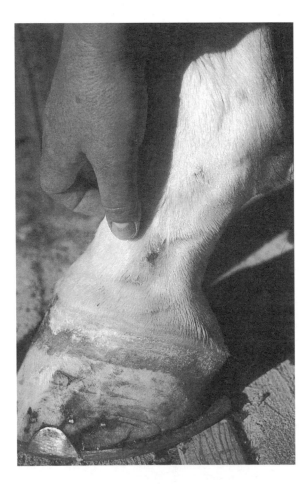

◀ WATCH FOR NICKS AND CUTS

If you spot some nicks and cuts in the fetlock or pastern area, as shown here, it probably indicates that your horse is hitting one leg with the other when he moves. This can be caused by having conformation that predisposes a horse to gait defects, being in poor condition, being young and uncoordinated, being shod improperly, slippery footing, or being worked fast or turned very sharply. If your horse tends to hit himself like this, you should determine if any of the above are causes and remedy the problems. You can also use protective boots on your horse during exercise. (See pp. 104–109.)

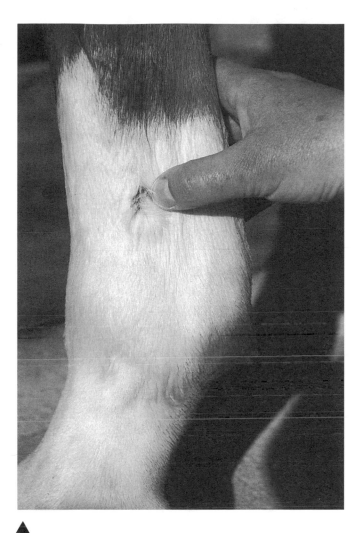

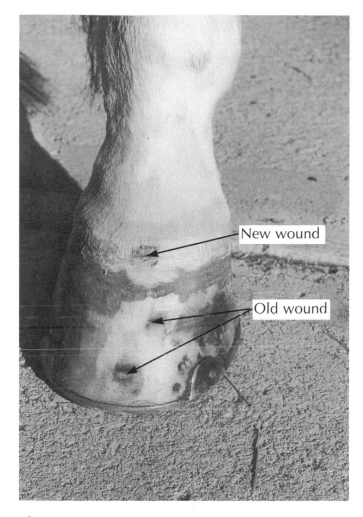

New wound

Old wound

WOUNDS FROM UNKNOWN CAUSES

A wound like this one that is higher up on the leg could have been caused by interference, but more likely it is one of the many nicks and scrapes a horse's leg receives over the years just from brush, fences, feeders, and unknown causes.

THE CORONARY BAND

When you are examining your horse's legs, be sure to look carefully at the coronary band, the junction of the skin and the hoof. A bruise or wound here can cause a horse to be lame and can affect hoof growth. Note that this horse shows multiple injuries. Besides the new wound on the coronary band, there is evidence of two others that have occurred and grown down. They can be seen as defects in the hoof wall. This horse needs proper conditioning and protective boots until this tendency disappears.

VITAL SIGNS

Vital signs are measurements of a horse's body functions and are a good indication of his overall state of health. You should learn how to take your horse's temperature, pulse, respiration, and measure capillary refill time, perform the pinch test, and become adept with a stethoscope for listening to the heart, lungs, and intestines. As with the daily check and leg check, vital signs will be much more meaningful if you first have normal values for each horse. Then, when your horse becomes ill, you can compare his vital signs with his previously established normals.

To establish normals, take the vital signs twice a day for three days and average the readings. Choose various times of day but always when the horse is at rest, not when he has just been working or is excited.

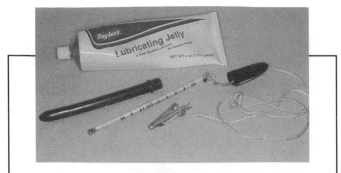

YOU WILL NEED an animal thermometer that has an eye in one end. Thread a string through the eye of the thermometer. On the other end of the string, tie a small alligator clip (found in hardware stores) or a spring-type clothespin. To make the thermometer easier to insert, use lubricating jelly (or petroleum jelly).

TAKING THE TEMPERATURE

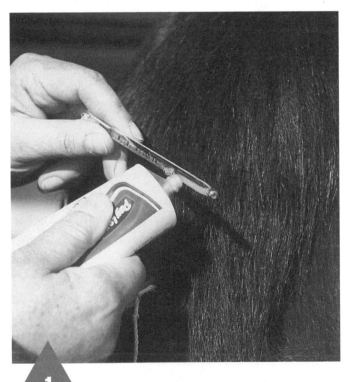

1 Check the thermometer to be sure it is reading below 96°F. If it registers a temperature from the previous use, hold it securely at the top and shake it sharply to get the mercury to drop down. Then apply a small amount of lubricating jelly to the business end of the thermometer. The lubricating jelly should be at room temperature, somewhere around 65°F.

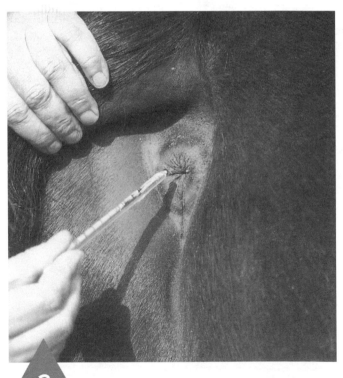

2 An assistant should be holding your horse, or your horse can be tied if he is used to having his temperature taken. Move your horse's tail off to one side. This tends to cause less tension in the horse than lifting the tail up. You will be inserting the thermometer into the anus at a slight upward angle, as shown here.

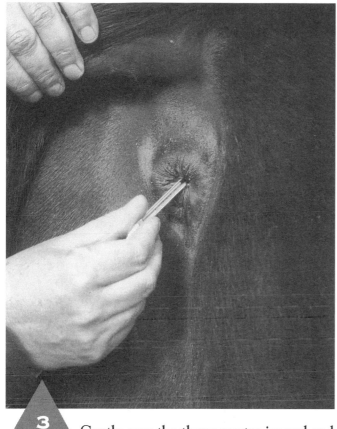

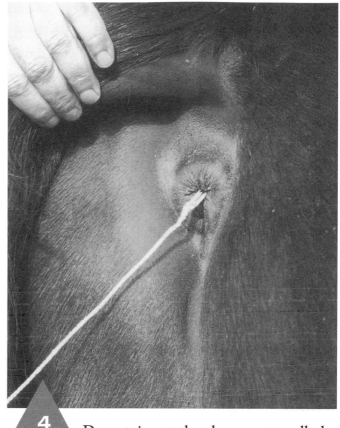

3 Gently ease the thermometer inward and upward until about 2 inches remains outside the anus.

4 Do not insert the thermometer all the way. If you do, it has a greater chance of contacting warm fecal material, which will give you an inaccurate temperature reading.

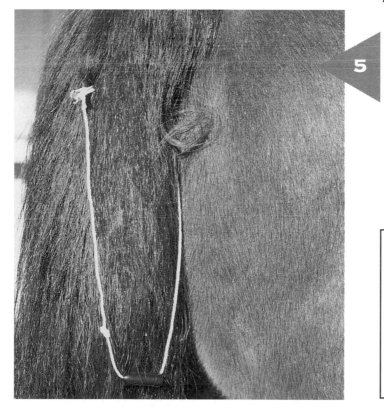

5 Move the tail back into position. Clip the string onto the horse's tail so that in case the horse defecates suddenly, the thermometer won't drop to the ground and break. The string will suspend it from the tail. After 2 minutes, take a reading. Wash your hands and the thermometer with antibacterial soap.

NORMAL TEMPERATURE

The range of average resting temperatures for adult horses is 99–100°F. Temperature increases with exertion, excitement, illness, and hot, humid weather. Temperature decreases with shock, and a horse's temperature can also be a few degrees lower in very cold weather.

TAKING A PULSE

You can take your horse's pulse just about any-where you can hear or feel his heartbeat. Here's how to determine pulse rate by palpation.

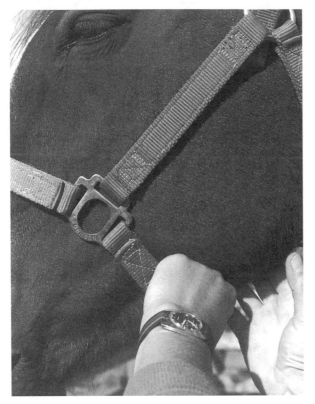

▲
PULSE ON MAXILLARY ARTERY

Choose an artery close to the surface of the skin. Lightly press your fingertips against the artery. Count the beats for 15 seconds and then multiply by 4 to get the rate per minute. The maxillary artery, on the inside of the jawbone, is one of the easiest places to find a strong pulse, even on a quiet, resting horse, such as this one. It's best not to let your thumb rest on the horse when you take a pulse as you might possibly pick up a throbbing from your own heartbeat and get a misreading.

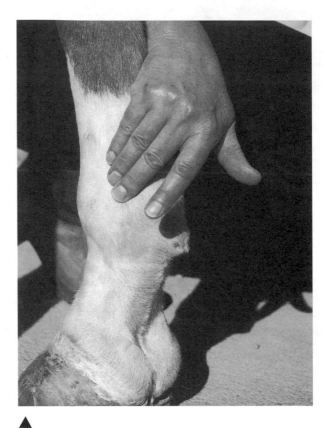

▲
PULSE ON DIGITAL ARTERY

Another easy-to-find pulse spot is the digital artery located on both the inside and outside of the horse's leg, just above the fetlock. On this horse, it is just under the middle finger.

NORMAL RESTING PULSE RATES
(IN BEATS PER MINUTE)

2 weeks old	up to 100
4 weeks old	70
Yearling	45–60
2 years old	40–50
Adult	30–40

Pulse rates are higher with excitement, pain, nervousness, elevated body temperature, shock, infectious disease, and exercise. Pulse rates are lower on fit horses and in cooler weather.

MEASURING RESPIRATION

A horse's normal resting respiration rate is usually between 12 and 25 breaths per minute. A foal's rate will be at the high end of the scale. One breath is measured as one inhalation and one exhalation. The ratio of the pulse to the respiration rate is often a more significant measure of stress than each of the actual figures is. Depending on the horse's age, his normal resting pulse to respiration ratio should range from 4:1 to 2:1. If the ratio becomes 1:1 or 1:2 (called inversion), the horse is suffering from oxygen deprivation, which indicates serious stress. Call your veterinarian immediately.

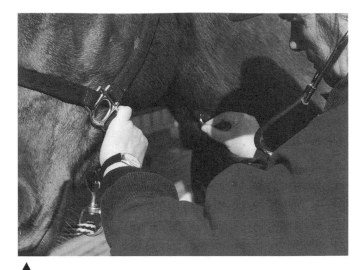

▲

USE A STETHOSCOPE ON THE TRACHEA
The best way to determine a respiration rate is to use a stethoscope on the trachea. With the earpieces forward, press the bell firmly into the underside of the horse's neck about 4 inches below the throatlatch. Count for 15 seconds, and multiply by 4.

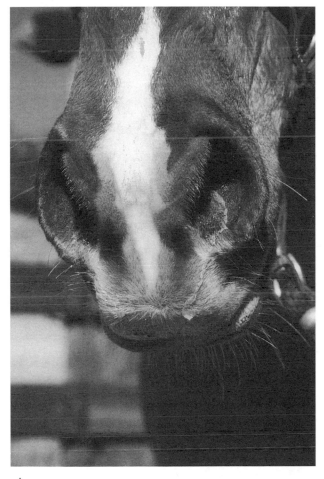

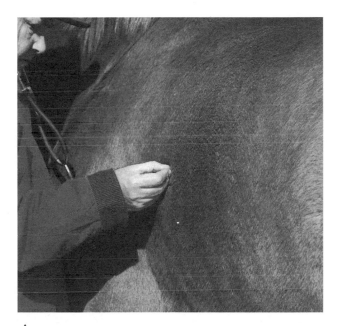

▲

WATCH THE HORSE'S NOSTRILS
When a horse is exercising heavily, it is easy to measure his respiration rate by watching his nostrils dilate and relax (each cycle counts as one breath) or by watching his ribs move in and out.

▲

USE A STETHOSCOPE ON THE LUNGS
Alternatively, you can listen to his lungs, but it takes more practice and experience to obtain a respiration rate this way. Place the stethoscope midway down the heart girth on the left side. You will hear the quality of the breathing process in his lungs but might not be able to identify definite breaths.

USING A STETHOSCOPE

Using a stethoscope can enable you to listen to your horse's respiratory tract, heart, and intestines. (See **Measuring Respiration** *to show how to listen to the air moving through the horse's trachea.) In all instances, the earpieces of the stethoscope should be worn forward. In most cases, the bell of the stethoscope must be pressed very firmly onto the horse in order for you to hear the sounds through the layers of hair, skin, and body tissue.*

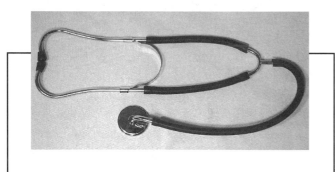

YOU CAN USE a stethoscope to listen to your horse's respiratory tract, heart, and intestines.

USING A STETHOSCOPE TO LISTEN TO THE HEART

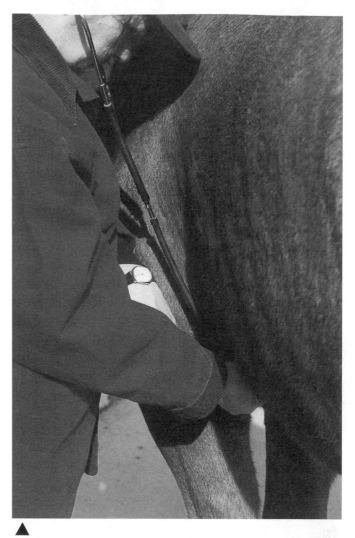

▲

To determine pulse or listen for heart function abnormalities, press the bell of the stethoscope into the horse's left (near side) armpit area. If you are using this method to take the pulse, count the heartbeat for 15 seconds and multiply by 4 to get the number of beats per minute.

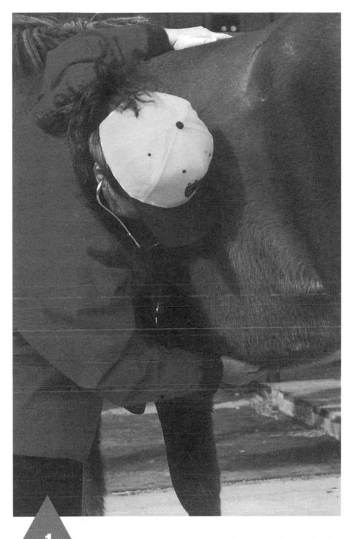

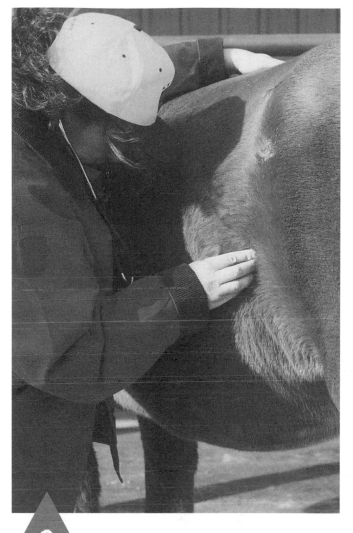

1 Select several sites on both sides of the horse. Steady the horse by placing your left hand on his back and using plenty of body-to-body contact with your left arm and shoulder. This way your horse won't be surprised when you place the bell of the stethoscope firmly into his belly as shown here. Become very familiar with what your horse's intestines normally sound like by spending 5 to 10 minutes for several days in a row listening to his gut both before and after he eats.

2 As you move the stethoscope to other locations on the abdomen, try to classify the nature of the sounds you hear to develop an ear for what is normal. Generally, you want to hear a moderate amount of gurgling, creaking, and swooshing. No sound could mean that the contents of your horse's intestines have become bound up (impacted), often from lack of proper moisture. Excessive gut sounds could be normal or could mean the horse has a hyperactive gut or diarrhea, such as might occur from a succulent pasture or rich alfalfa hay.

PERFORMNG A PINCH TEST

The pinch test is a quick and easy subjective way to evaluate skin turgor (normal state of distention and resiliency) and measure dehydration. However, the best indication that your horse is properly hydrated is to know that he is drinking plenty of fresh water and that his manure is moist.

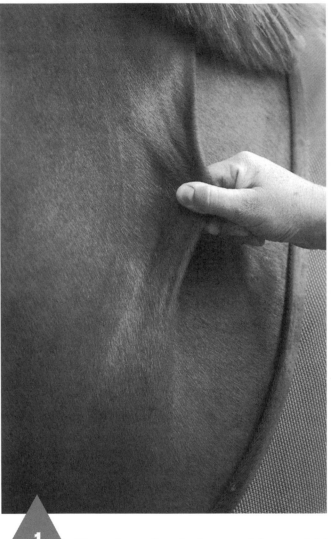

1 To perform the pinch test, pick up a fold of skin in the neck/shoulder area and pull it away from the horse's body.

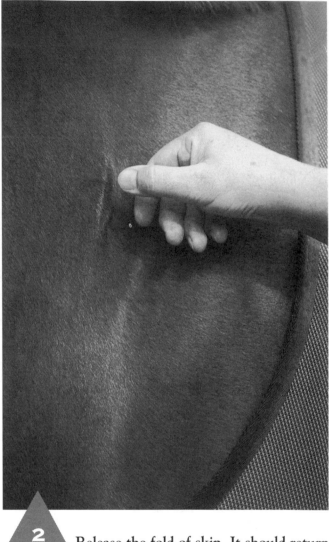

2 Release the fold of skin. It should return almost immediately to its normal flat position.

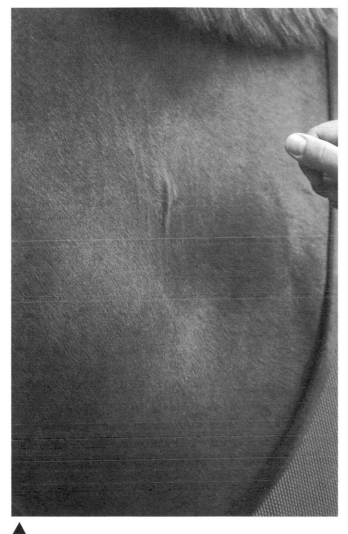

▲ NORMAL

This is acceptable and normal for this horse during winter: showing the fold of skin 2 seconds after release. If the skin remains markedly peaked for 2 to 3 seconds, it probably indicates a degree of body fluid loss. A "standing tent" of skin of a 5- to 10-second duration indicates moderate to severe dehydration that might require the attention of your veterinarian.

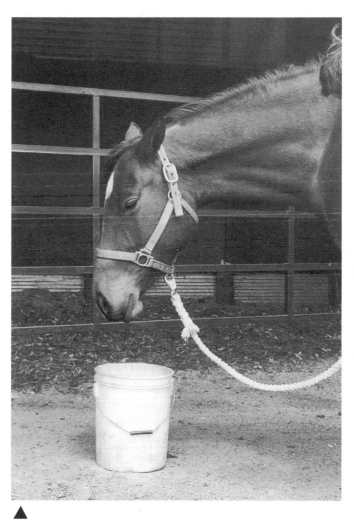

▲ WARNING SIGN

If your horse is dehydrated but refuses to drink, it might be an indication that his electrolytes are imbalanced and his normal thirst response is not working.

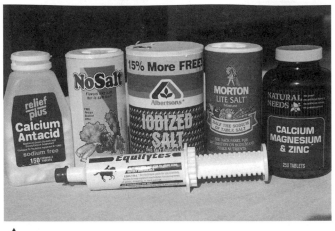

▲

ELECTROLYTES

Electrolytes are minerals that are necessary for many body functions. A horse normally gets all of the electrolytes he requires from good quality hay and a calcium-phosphorus trace mineral salt block. However, sometimes it is necessary to provide electrolytes along with water to get a dehydrated horse back on track. There are various commercial equine electrolyte formulas on the market, such as the one in the foreground of this photo. Be sure you read all of the ingredients carefully and confer with your veterinarian to make sure you use the appropriate formula for your horse's specific condition.

Electrolytes can also be provided using some items you might have around the house. Back row from the left: sodium-free calcium antacid; No Salt, which is 100% potassium chloride; iodized salt, which is sodium chloride with iodine added; Lite Salt, which is 50% sodium chloride and 50% potassium chloride; and calcium, magnesium, and zinc tablets. If a horse is eating alfalfa hay, he probably does not need calcium supplements.

PROVIDING ELECTROLYTE SUPPLEMENTS

Here are a few recipes that you could use to provide your horse with electrolytes. For a horse in hard work that sweats a lot, is fed alfalfa hay, and requires sodium, chloride, and potassium supplements in the correct proportion on a regular basis, give 1–4 tablespoons per day in the feed or water:

✦ 3 parts regular table salt
✦ 1 part No Salt (potassium chloride)

For a horse that has just worked hard, is on a diet of grass hay, and requires immediate supplements, fill an old dewormer syringe (that you have washed out thoroughly) and give your horse the following homemade paste:

✦ 3 tablespoons regular table salt
✦ 1 tablespoon No Salt
✦ 2 tablets sodium-free calcium antacid (crushed)
✦ 2 250 mg magnesium tablets (crushed)
✦ Flavoring such as honey, molasses, syrup, applesauce

MEASURING CAPILLARY REFILL TIME

You can get more information on your horse's over-all health and the function of his circulatory system by inspecting the mucous membranes around his eyes and gums. They should be a bright pink color and appropriately moist. If the mucous membranes are very pale or white, the horse is suffering from a blood loss or circulatory impairment. If the gums are bright red, it indicates a toxic (poison) condition. If the gums look a grayish blue color, the horse is probably in shock.

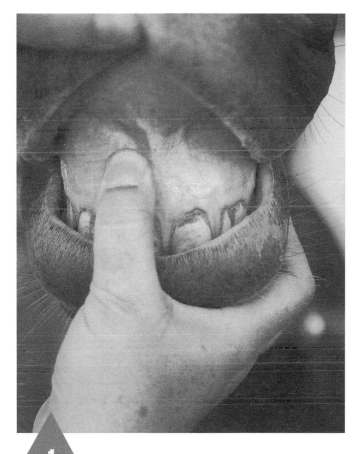

1 With your horse haltered and an assistant holding him, roll back the horse's upper lip with your left hand. With your right hand on the lower jaw, exert thumb pressure on the gum above the upper incisors for about 2 seconds. This will blanch (squeeze the blood temporarily out of the capillaries) a spot on the gum.

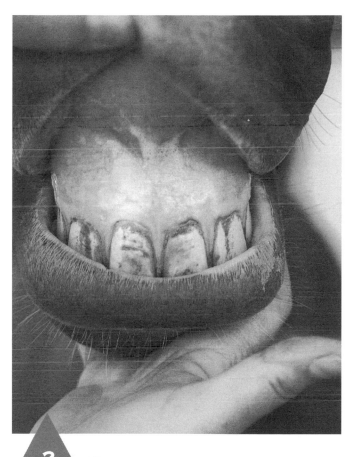

2 When you remove your thumb, a circular white spot will remain. Within 1 second, the spot should return to its original color. This is the "capillary refill time." If it takes 5 to 10 seconds for the color to return, your horse is showing signs of circulatory impairment. Extended capillary refill time is often seen in horses with severe colic or those that are in shock.

Dental Care

TOOTH ERUPTION

Horses have incisors, premolars, and molars. There are 12 incisors at the front of the mouth, 12 premolars beginning at the corner of the lips, and 12 molars at the back of the mouth. Premolar does not refer to a temporary tooth but to a position of the tooth in the mouth. Premolars are teeth in front of the molars. In between the premolars and the incisors, there is a relatively toothless space called the interdental space. However, male horses have four canine teeth in the interdental space and some horses have wolf teeth in front of the premolars.

Before a horse gets his permanent teeth, he gets a set of temporary teeth. For example, the temporary premolars are in place by 2 weeks of age but are replaced by the permanent premolars between the ages of 2 and 5 years. Unfortunately, the numbering system for premolars is confusing due to the wolf tooth being called the permanent 1st premolar. The 1st deciduous premolar is replaced by the 2nd permanent premolar, and so on.

Wolf teeth are permanent teeth but sometimes they are pushed out (along with the temporary 1st premolar) when the 2nd permanent premolar erupts at 2 to 3 years of age. Other times, the wolf teeth are removed by the veterinarian.

DECIDUOUS ("BABY" OR TEMPORARY) TOOTH ERUPTION

TOOTH	AGE TOOTH APPEARS
1st incisor	Birth
2nd incisor	4–6 weeks
3rd incisor	6–9 months
1st premolar	2 weeks
2nd premolar	2 weeks
3rd premolar	2 weeks

WOLF TEETH

Through evolutionary processes, the first premolars, also called "wolf teeth," are absent in some horses. Usually, if a horse does have wolf teeth, it will be a pair of upper wolf teeth and they will have erupted by the time he is a yearling. Wolf teeth can sometimes cause painful pinching of the lip skin when a snaffle bit is used on the horse. Because of this, wolf teeth are often extracted.

PERMANENT TOOTH ERUPTION

TOOTH	AGE TOOTH APPEARS
1st incisor (replaces 1st deciduous incisor)	2½ years
2nd incisor (replaces 2nd deciduous incisor)	3½ years
3rd incisor (replaces 3rd deciduous incisor)	4½ years
Canines (in male horses and a few mares)	4–5 years
1st premolar (wolf teeth)	5–6 months
2nd premolar (replaces 1st deciduous premolar)	2–3 years
3rd premolar (replaces 2nd deciduous premolar)	3–4 years
4th premolar (replaces 3rd deciduous premolar)	4–5 years
1st molar	9–12 months
2nd molar	2 years
3rd molar	3½–4 years

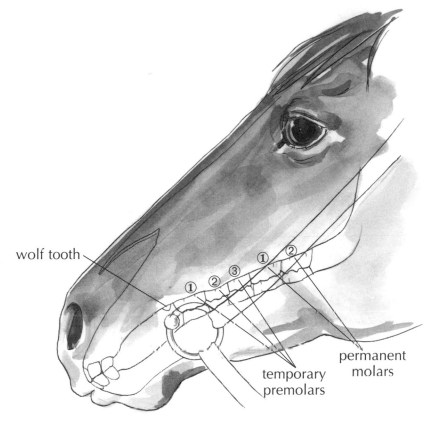

wolf tooth

temporary premolars

permanent molars

◄ TWO-YEAR-OLD HORSE

This shows the teeth of a 2-year-old horse. Note that the incisors are small deciduous teeth. There is a permanent first premolar (wolf tooth) present. Temporary premolars 1–3 are in place as well as permanent molars #1 and 2. Permanent molar #3, which will erupt at the rear of the jaw, will appear at age 3½–4.

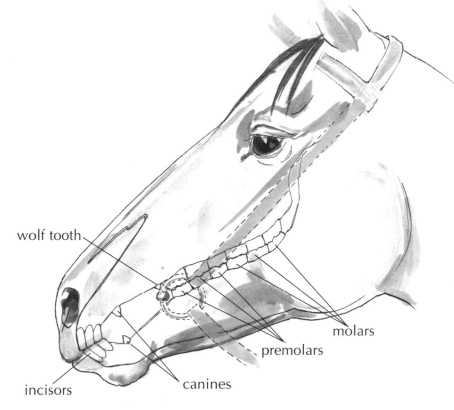

wolf tooth

molars

premolars

incisors

canines

◄ MATURE MALE HORSE

This shows the teeth of a mature male horse. Note that the canines have already emerged, all of the permanent molars and premolars are present, and that a wolf tooth is present.

THE HORSE'S JAW

Male horses have an additional set of teeth called "canines" or "tushes" that are located behind the incisors. Male canines usually begin to erupt at 4 years of age and are usually fully developed at 5. Canines can get very sharp and usually need to be clipped or rasped. A very few mares develop tiny canine buds.

Until a horse is 5 years old, his teeth are constantly erupting, shedding, and being replaced. When a horse is 5, he is said to be aged and have a full set of teeth. However, a horse's teeth continue to emerge until he is in his early 20s.

The upper jaw of a horse is 30% wider than the lower jaw. As the horse grinds his food with a sideways motion, he wears his molars down and sharp edges form on the outside (cheek surfaces) of the upper molars and premolars and on the inside (tongue surfaces) of his lower molars and premolars.

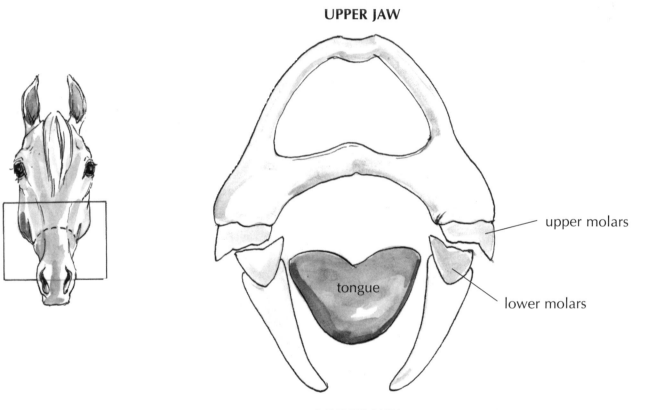

UPPER JAW

upper molars

tongue

lower molars

LOWER JAW

An inside view of the horse's mouth showing the need for *floating*. Because the upper jaw is wider than the lower jaw, sharp points form on the outside edge (cheek surface) of the upper molars and the inside edge (tongue surface) of the lower molars. These need to be filed off regularly.

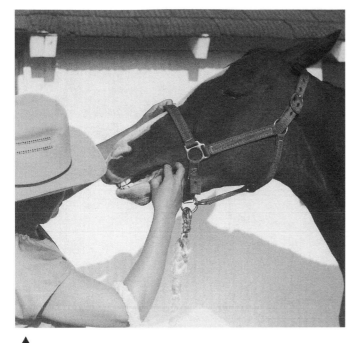

▲
EXAMINING YOUR HORSE'S MOUTH

Become familiar with your horse's mouth so you can tell when things are abnormal. Periodically inspect the gums, tongue, and sharpness of the teeth. It is natural for a horse to raise his head like this when you are handling his mouth. In fact, it makes it easier for you to get a good look. Before you examine your horse's mouth, loosen his halter a few notches so it will be easier for him to open his mouth. It is natural for a horse to chew and work his tongue while his mouth is being examined. His tongue is a very strong muscle and his jaws are designed to crush and grind dry grains.

DENTAL WARNING SIGNS

If your horse shows any of these signs, he may be asking for a dental appointment:

✦ If he drops wads of feed while eating

✦ If there is hay and grain in the water bucket

✦ If he holds his head at an odd angle while chewing

✦ If he doesn't eat

✦ If he is in poor condition

✦ If he has a very bad mouth odor

✦ If he tosses or shakes his head when wearing a bridle

✦ If he roots his nose up into the air when you apply pressure with the bridle reins

✦ If he resists turning one way or the other

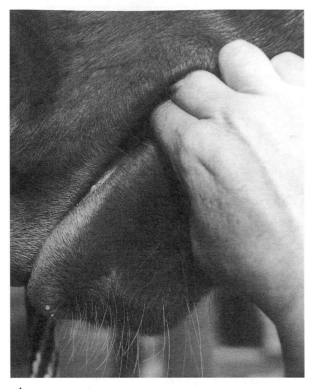

▲
Know the Interdental Space

It is important to know where you can and cannot place your hands. Learn where the safe interdental space is by inserting two fingers in your horse's mouth about at the corner of his lips. Be careful — in some horses, this might put your fingers pretty close to the premolars.

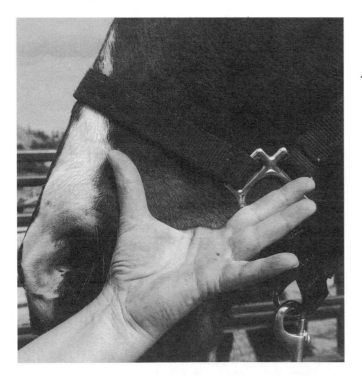

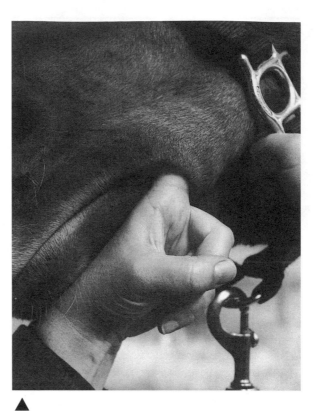

▲
Approach the Premolars

Insert your index finger between the cheek and teeth. Pull outward on the cheek tissue so that your finger is a safe distance from the molars. If you accidentally get your finger between the upper and lower teeth, your horse's powerful jaws could break or sever your finger. Relax the outward pull on the cheek tissue and begin approaching the edge of the premolars.

◀ ## Feel for Sharp Edges

I find that with my palm outward, I can more safely feel for sharp edges. By the way, if a horse has not had his teeth floated for some time, his teeth can be so sharp that they can cut your finger. Teeth that sharp can also cut the inside of his cheeks.

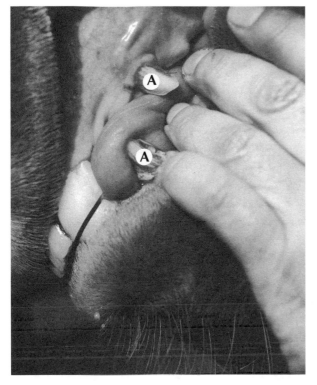

▲
SHARP CANINES

This 6-year-old gelding has sharp points on his canines (A). These could hurt his tongue, particularly if his mouth were held shut with a noseband. These sharp points should be filed smooth. This gelding has not yet formed a corner hook — his corner incisor is still flat-surfaced. The corner incisor shows no sign of Galvayne's Groove (compare with the following photo).

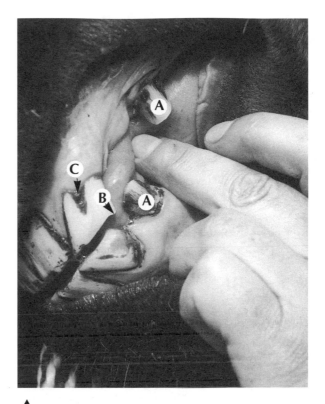

▲
FILED CANINES

This 12-year-old gelding has had his canines (A) filed so they have a flat, rounded surface. (Compare these to the sharp ones above at left.) This older gelding has a *hook* on his corner (3rd) incisor (B), a tooth feature that appears when the horse is 7 years old, then disappears at 9 and reappears in some instances at 11.

If the hook can appear at 7 and again at 11, how would you know how old this gelding is? Look at the dark, V-shaped groove at the gum line of the corner incisor (C). This is called *Galvayne's Groove*. In this horse, it is filled with food material, which makes it easier to see. In many horses, the groove appears at age 10, is halfway down the tooth by age 15, and will reach the bottom of the tooth by age 20. At age 25, the groove will have disappeared from the top half of the tooth, and at age 30 it will be gone from the entire tooth. So you know this horse is over 10, but not yet 15.

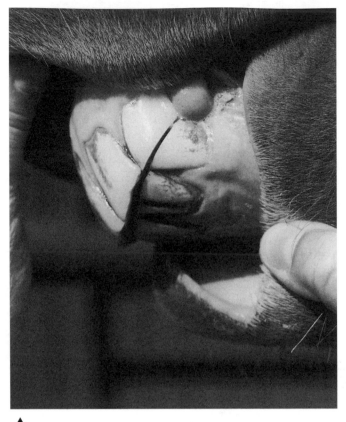

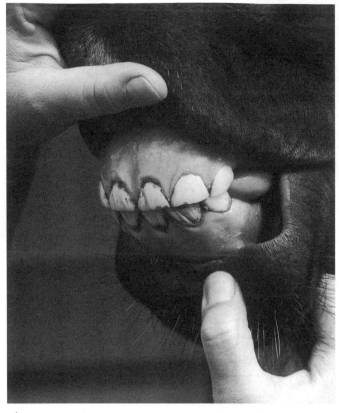

PARROT MOUTH

It is desirable for the incisors to meet evenly. This 6-year-old gelding has a slight overbite, which is called a *parrot mouth*. A severe overbite could prevent a horse from grazing efficiently. It is avoided in breeding stock since the condition is considered hereditary. If you are showing your stallion or mare in a halter or conformation class, the judge may ask you to part the horse's lips like this so he or she can see if the horse's teeth meet evenly.

OVERBITE

This 2-year-old filly has a slight overbite. Notice the difference in size between these temporary "baby" or "milk" teeth as compared to the adult incisors in the previous photos.

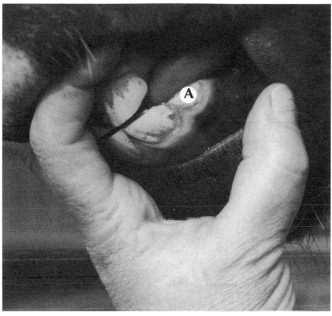

▲

CUTTING TEETH

This 8-month-old weanling colt is just "cutting" his temporary (3rd) corner incisors (A). The lower one is about halfway in; the upper one hasn't started coming in yet. When a young horse is cutting teeth, he may chew on things as a way to relieve his sore gums. This is one reason young horses frequently chew wood, metal, lead ropes, and anything else they can get their teeth on.

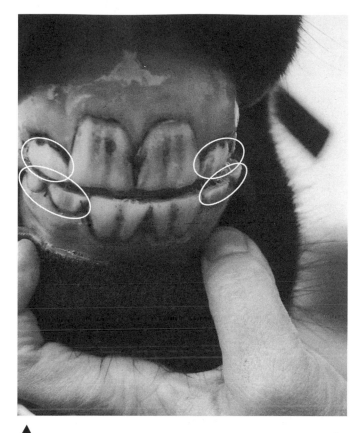

▲

CENTRAL INCISORS

This 3-year-old filly still has eight of her temporary incisors (circled), but she has her permanent four central incisors. Note the size difference between the temporary and permanent teeth.

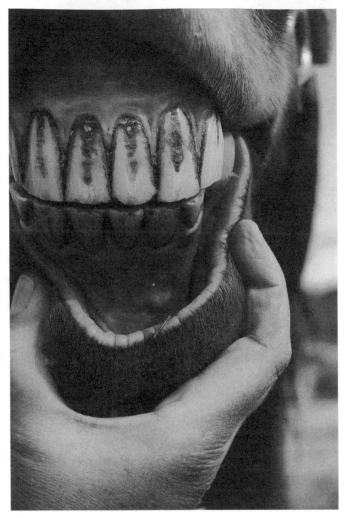

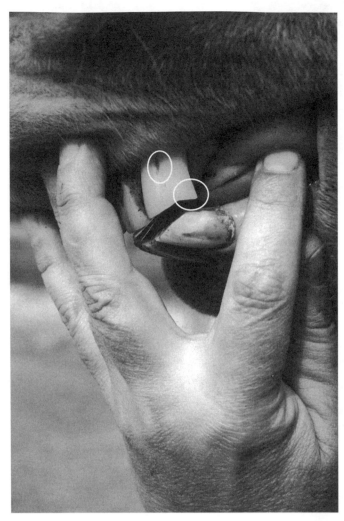

20-YEAR-OLD MARE (FRONT)
This shows the incisors of a very healthy, 20-year-old mare. Note that the gums tend to recede with age.

20-YEAR-OLD MARE (SIDE)
The same 20-year-old mare's teeth from the side show how the incisors tend to angle forward more with age. Also note the corner "hook" that reappeared at age 11 and is still here at age 20. Notice that this 20-year-old mare did not "read the book" when it comes to Galvayne's Groove because it is only about halfway down her top corner incisor, more like it would be on a 15-year-old horse. (You can see this in the previous photo as well.)

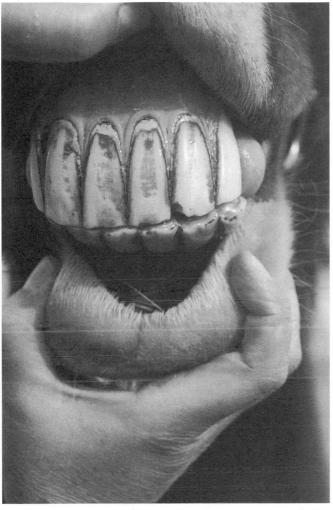

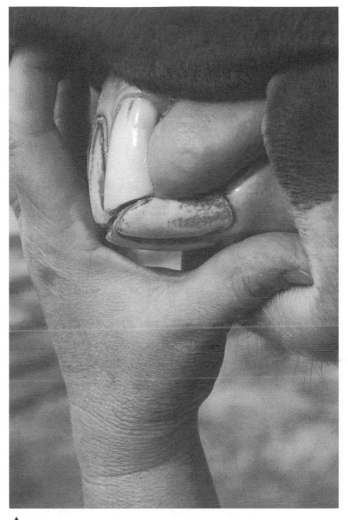

▲
19-YEAR-OLD MARE (FRONT)

This shows the incisors of a 19-year-old mare that had a broken lower jaw as a young horse, which off-set her lower jaw to her upper jaw and caused her to lose three permanent premolars. All of this has caused her to have more than her share of dental problems. She appears to be very "long in the tooth" when compared to her 20-year-old herdmate in the previous photos. She has a tartar buildup along the gum line.

▲
19-YEAR-OLD MARE (SIDE)

The same 19-year-old mare. Note that her lower incisors show extreme elongation; they are almost horizontal. This mare did not redevelop the corner hook at age 11 or 12. And there is no evidence of Galvayne's Groove on either of her corner incisors. Comparing her to "the book" and her herdmate of a similar age just goes to show that although certain dental rules apply to many equines, you must take all circumstances into consideration when interpreting what you see.

Genital Care

WASHING THE MARE'S PERINEAL AREA

Whether you are preparing a mare for breeding or foaling or just practicing good overall hygiene, periodically you will need to wash the mare's perineal area.

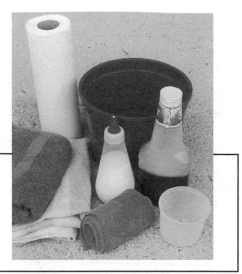

YOU WILL NEED a tail wrap, warm water, a small pail, a splash cup, mild regular soap or antibacterial soap (depending on whether it's a routine or a pre-reproductive wash), absorbent terrycloth towels, and paper towels. Some people are more comfortable if they wear rubber or surgical gloves when washing the genitals.

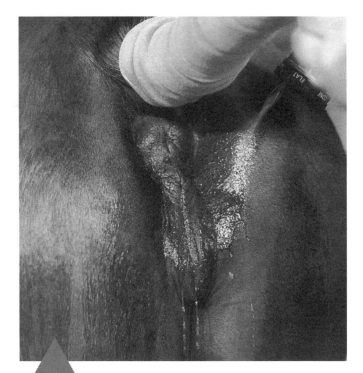

1 Wrap the mare's tail to raise it out of the way. If you are washing before breeding or foaling, the mare's tail should be completely encased in a tube sock or other wrapping. Wet the mare's rectal and genital area *indirectly* with a gentle spray of *warm* water. If you use a forceful spray, it could send debris into the vagina. If you use cold water, it will probably cause the mare to display a sudden reaction that is part of the croup and perineal reflex chains. She might clamp her tail, drop her hindquarters, and squat toward the ground. If she is very sensitive and unfamiliar with the process, cold water could make her kick or buck — so use warm water.

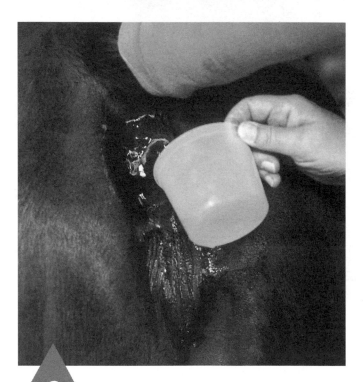

2 Wet the perineal area before soaping. This flushes away large particles of debris and softens the material that has adhered to the external tissues. If you don't have direct access to warm water in a hose, carry a bucket from the house and use the splash cup to wet the perineal area.

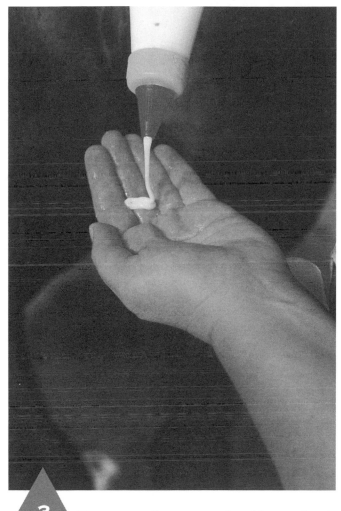

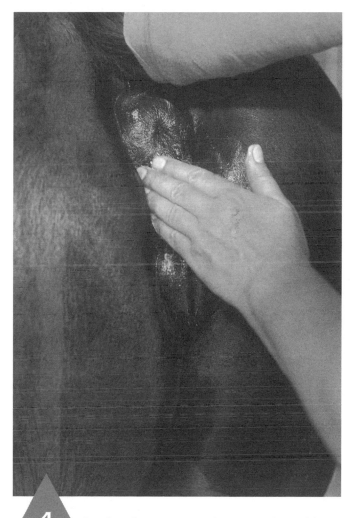

3 Place a small amount of mild soap (such as Ivory Soap, not detergent) on your hand. This is the maximum that should be used. Close and open your fist a couple of times to distribute the soap evenly over your palm and fingers.

4 Apply the soap with a gentle rubbing motion, taking care not to open the labia (lips) of the vulva. Your goal is to clean the external organs without contaminating the internal portion of the mare's reproductive tract. Wash from the center of the perineal area outward.

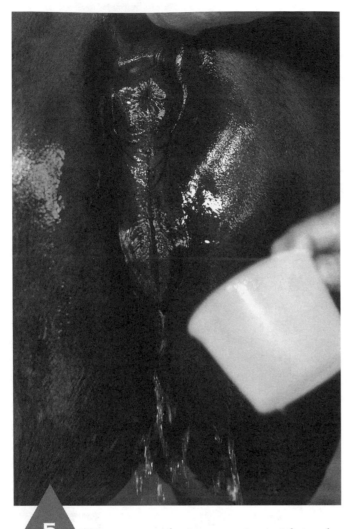

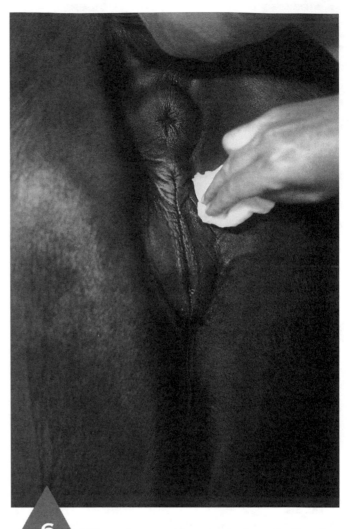

5 Rinse several times, using either the splash cup or a gentle, indirect mist from the hose. After one round of rinsing, you may want to gently rub the entire area you washed and then rinse some more. If you are preparing a mare for breeding, palpation, or foaling, you should follow this initial cleansing wash with two sequences using antibacterial soap.

6 Wipe the mare's external genitalia dry using disposable paper towels. Wipe from the median line outward. Do not wipe across the vulvar opening.

CLEANING THE MALE'S SHEATH

Male horses might have difficulty urinating or might rub their tails because of a dirty sheath. The sheath is the protective envelope of skin around the penis. Fatty secretions, dead skin cells, and dirt accumulate in the folds of the sheath. This black, foul smelling, somewhat waxy substance is called smegma. Depending on the individual horse's smegma production, the sheath should be cleaned about once or twice a year. You can clean the sheath somewhat with the penis retracted into the sheath, but you can do a more thorough job if the penis is down. Once a horse is accustomed to the procedure, he will likely relax and let his penis down for cleaning. Usually the best time for this is on a warm day after a workout when the horse is somewhat tired and relaxed. If the horse is very touchy in his genital area, you could have your veterinarian tranquilize the horse so your horse will be more manageable and relaxed.

ANATOMY OF THE SHEATH OF THE MALE HORSE

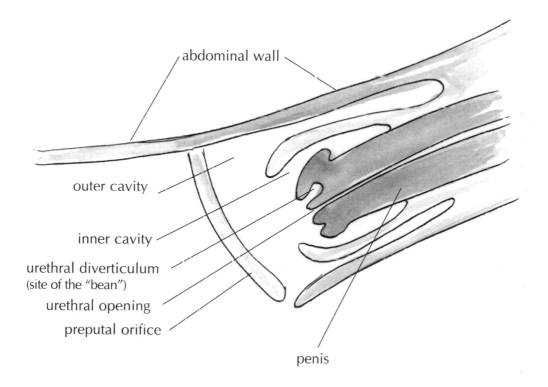

Note the folds of skin that can trap debris and smegma. Also note the site of "bean" formation, the *diverticulum* (blind pouch) adjacent to the urethral opening.

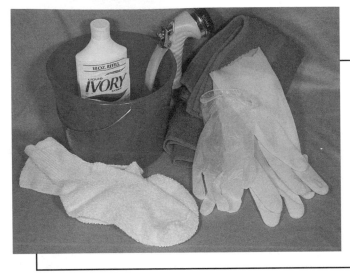

YOU WILL NEED warm water, a hose, a small bucket, mild soap, rubber gloves, a tube sock, and hand towels.

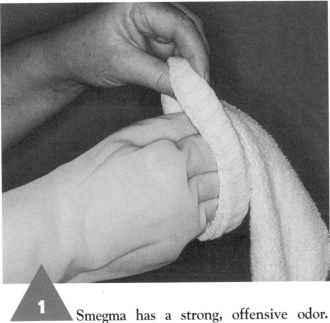

1 Smegma has a strong, offensive odor. Before you clean the sheath, first put a rubber glove on your right hand.

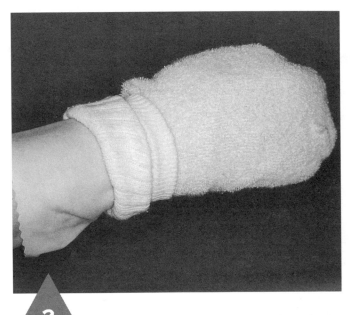

2 Cover your gloved hand with a large tube sock.

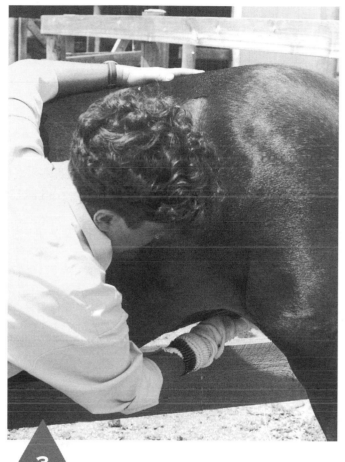

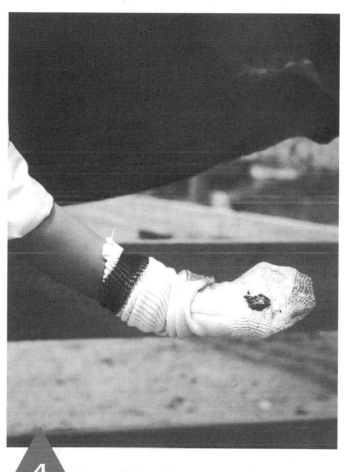

▲3 Use a safe handling position with your left hand up on the horse's back. Do not lower your head to see what you are doing or you could be kicked. Soak the sock in warm water and wet the sheath area with water. Add a very small amount of liquid soap (such as Ivory) to the tube sock and begin washing the sheath inside and out. (There are also several commercial products designed especially for sheath cleaning.)

▲4 You will be able to remove large chunks and sheets of smegma as you work.

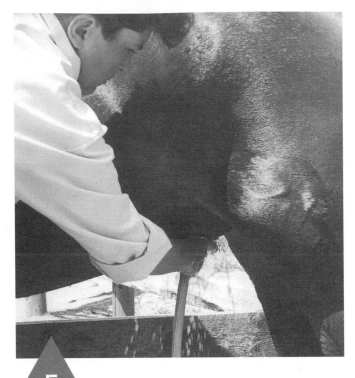

5 ► The best way I have found to rinse the sheath thoroughly is to use a hose, warm water, and moderate to low pressure. Most horses learn to tolerate, then enjoy, this after one session. You can insert the hose 2 to 3 inches into the sheath to rinse.

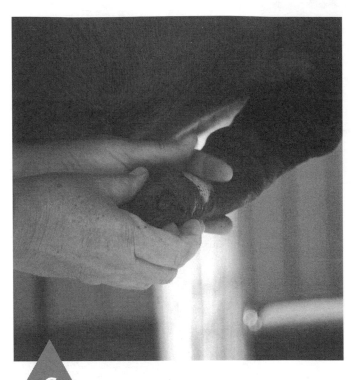

6 ► Often a ball of smegma, called a *bean*, will accumulate in the diverticulum near the urethral opening. The bean can build up to a size that could interfere with urination. Sometimes the bean material is white. To remove it, move the skin at the end of the penis near the urethral opening until you find a blind pouch. This part of sheath cleaning is when your horse is most likely to kick.

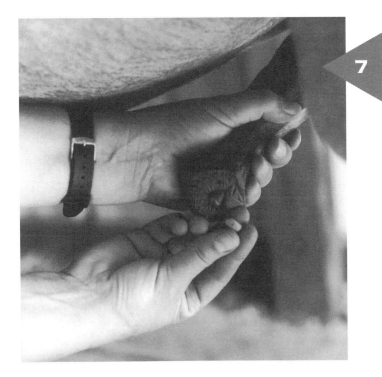

7 ◄ Usually you can roll the bean out quite easily. This bean is of a size and hardness that could cause discomfort on urination.

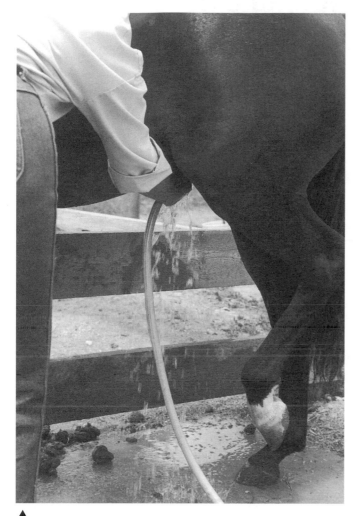

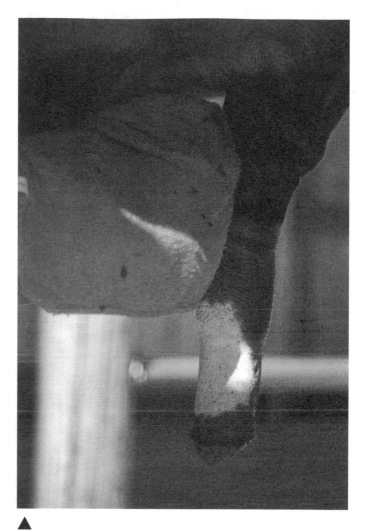

▲
CAUTION

Until he becomes accustomed to having his sheath cleaned, a horse's natural reaction is to kick upward with one of the hind legs. A horse can easily reach a fly on his belly with this method, so your right hand and arm could be in danger. Hold them as high and as close to the horse's belly as possible until the horse gets used to the sensation of the water.

▲
OLDER HORSES

Older horses that are quite used to the process will lower the penis so you can clean the penis also. Use only warm water on the penis — no soap.

Protecting a Horse from Pests and Parasites

DEWORMING

All horses have worms. Your job is to keep them under control with good sanitation, manure removal, bot egg removal, and deworming. Your deworming program should target strongyles (bloodworms), ascarids (roundworms), Oxyuris equi (pinworms), and Gasterophilus (bots). Adult horses should be dewormed every two months, year-round. Foals should be dewormed from one month of age, every month until they are weaned, then every six weeks until they are one year old. After that they can join the adult program of six times a year.

At least twice a year, use a product such as ivermectin that is effective against all worms and bots. There are two strategic times to use a bot dewormer. One is during early spring (April or May, depending on your climate), just before bot larvae leave the horse's stomach. The other is in late fall, after a killing frost and after all bot eggs have been removed from the horse's coat (October or November, depending on your climate). The other four times, you can also use ivermectin or you can choose from other dewormers, paying close attention to their effectiveness against strongyles, which are the biggest parasite threat to your horse's health.

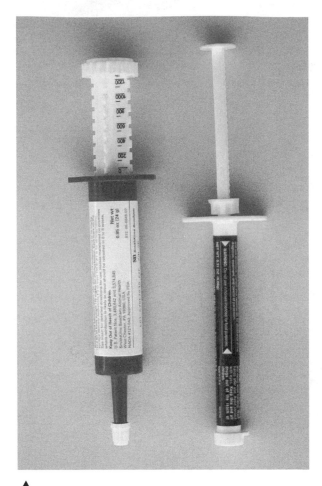
▲

PASTE DEWORMER

The easiest and most effective way to deworm your horse is to use paste dewormer in a tube. Most equine dewormers are either a low-volume dose (about 6 ml) or a high-volume dose (about 20 ml). Most ivermectin products are a low-volume dose. Low-volume dewormers are easier to administer: There is less to insert in the horse's mouth so there is less chance for mess and waste, and the smaller syringes are easier for small hands to operate one-handed. Dewormers should be at a low room temperature when administered. If they are too cold, they can be stiff and difficult to dispense from the tube. If they are too warm, they won't stick to the horse's tongue and palate well. Check the expiration date on the dewormer box or tube. Be sure you use a fresh product.

SAMPLE SCHEDULE	
January 1	Dewormer
March 1	Dewormer
May 1	Dewormer plus boticide
July 1	Dewormer
September 1	Dewormer
November 1	Dewormer plus boticide

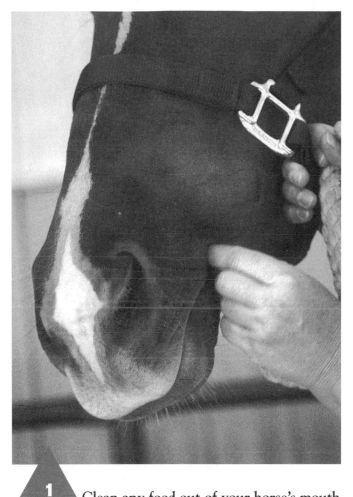

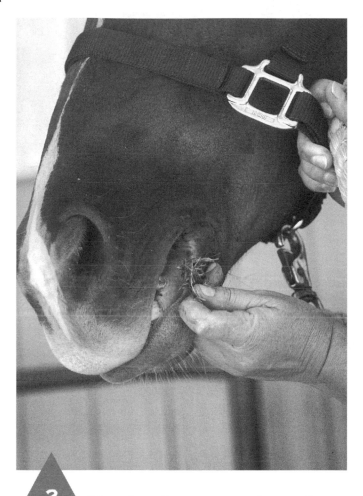

1 Clean any food out of your horse's mouth so that your horse does not mix the dewormer with the food and spit it out. If you are working alone, you can hold the lead rope and the cheek portion of the halter with your right hand and clean out the mouth with your left hand. Insert your fingers at the corners of your horse's lips and enter the interdental space where there are no teeth. (See p. 30.)

2 Often just the presence of your fingers will cause your horse to begin moving his tongue and jaw and drop any hay wads he has hidden in the recesses of his mouth. Other times you will have to reach into the safe zones to remove wads of feed.

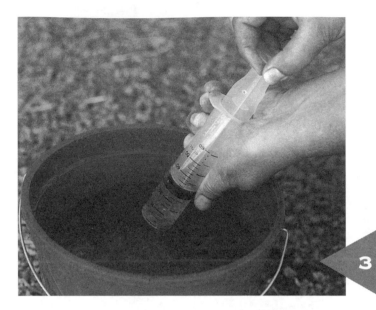

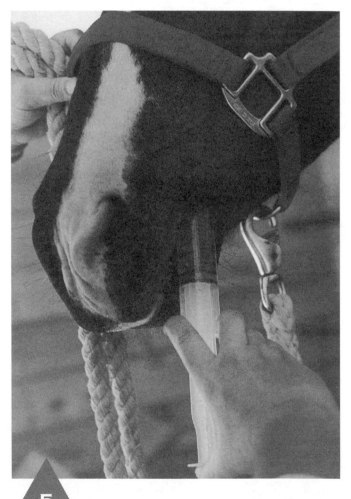

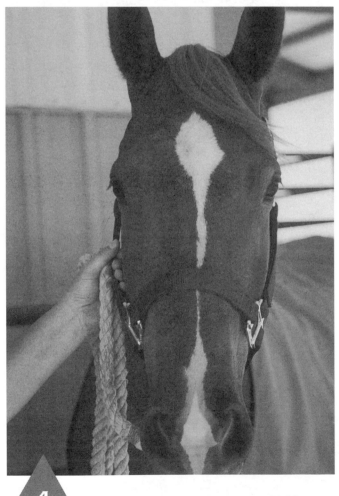

3 To further clean your horse's mouth, flush it out with warm water. Remove the needle from a 60 cc plastic syringe and fill it with warm water.

4 If you have an assistant to hold your horse, things will be even easier. But since you may need to perform routine deworming alone, I will show you the solo method. Hold the lead rope and the cheek piece of the horse's halter with your left hand.

5 You may find you have more control if you slide your hand over to the noseband instead. Insert the syringe full of water into the corner of your horse's mouth between his teeth and his cheek.

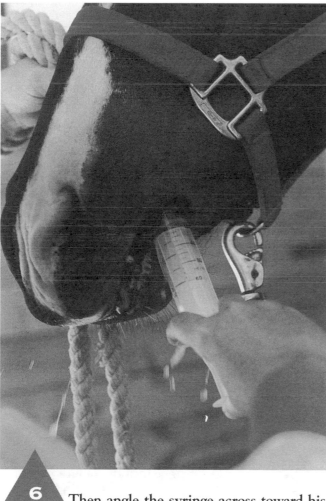

6 Then angle the syringe across toward his tongue and depress the plunger, releasing the water into his mouth. You may need to flush with two or three syringes of water if your horse's mouth was particularly full of food.

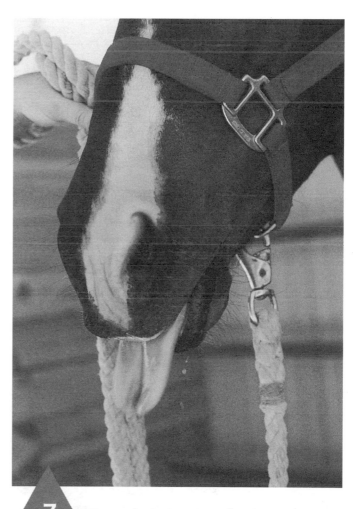

7 Wait a few minutes in order to let him work all of the water out of his mouth before you proceed. The dewormer won't stick to a very wet tongue or palate.

USING LOW-VOLUME DOSE DEWORMER

Determine your horse's weight (see **Measuring Weight**, *p. 59).*

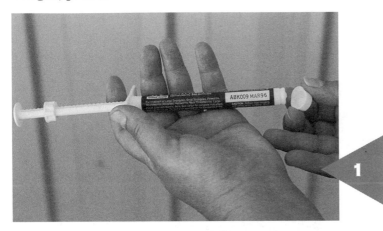

1 Adjust the syringe to the proper dosage according to your horse's weight. Remove the cap from the syringe. Note the clearly marked expiration date on the label. Always be sure to use a fresh product.

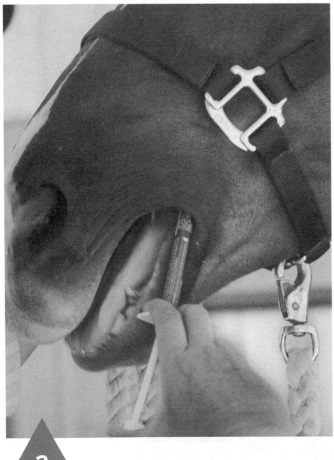

2 Use the same basic procedure to administer the dewormer as you did for flushing the mouth. With the halter (or the noseband) in your left hand and the syringe in your right hand, insert the tube at an upward angle between the horse's premolars and cheek.

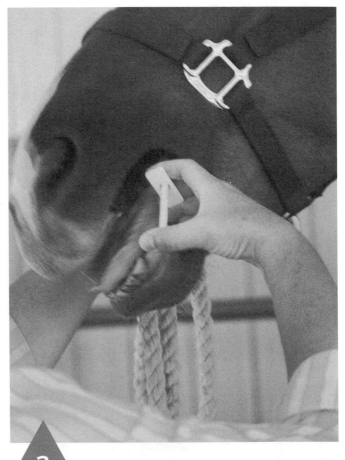

3 Turn the syringe into the mouth cavity. If you are deworming a horse that opens his mouth and works his tongue right away, you'll be better off applying the dewormer to the *roof* of his mouth. If you apply it onto a busy tongue, he will likely spit it out as soon as you apply it.

USING HIGH-VOLUME DOSE DEWORMER

Determine your horse's weight (see **Measuring Body Weight,** *p. 59).*

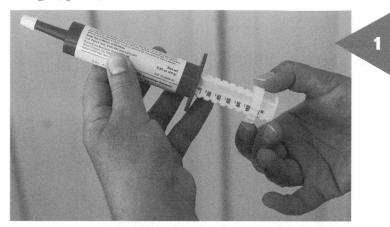

1 Adjust the syringe to the proper dosage according to your horse's weight. Lock the ring into position so when you depress the plunger, it will stop dispensing at the desired dosage.

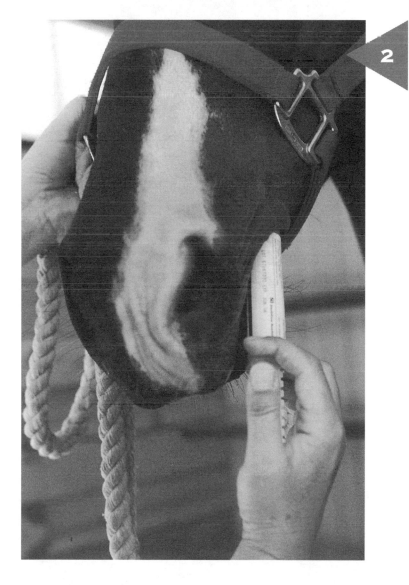

2 If you are deworming a quiet-mouthed horse, insert the large tube just a few inches.

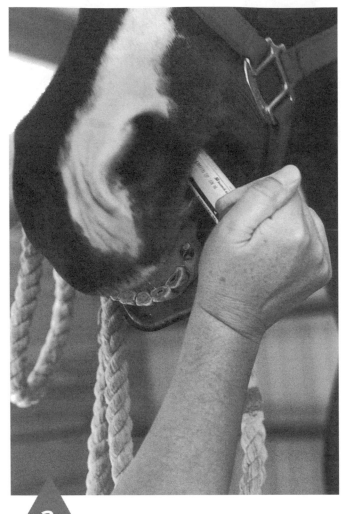

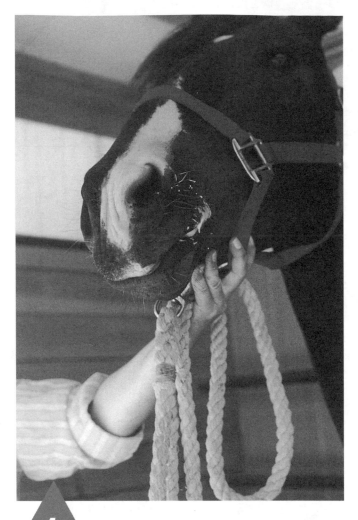

▲3 Turn the dewormer tube inward and dispense the product onto the tongue. If the dewormer was at low room temperature, it will dispense easily.

▲4 It is always a good idea, but especially if you are using a high-volume dose, to hold the horse's head up for a minute so the dewormer has time to dissolve in his mouth.

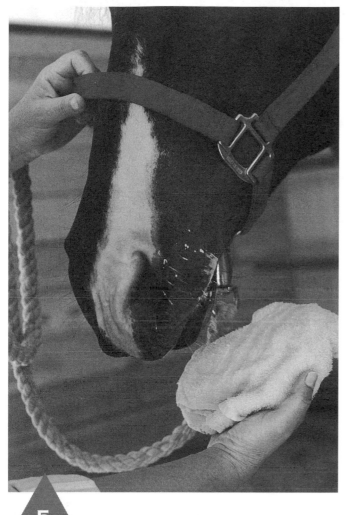

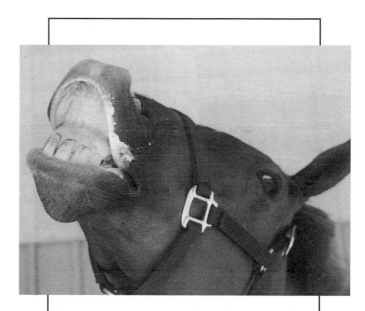

5 If some dewormer has ended up on your horse's lips (this seems to be more common with high-volume dewormer), wipe it off with a damp cloth.

FLEHMEN RESPONSE

Some horses exhibit the Flehmen response, which is a reaction to odd smells or tastes. The horse curls up his upper lip and raises his head. It is a comical, individual response of some horses, perfectly normal for them and nothing to worry about.

REMOVING BOT EGGS

Gasterophilus, *commonly called bots, are a parasite that have the following life cycle. A bot fly (which looks like a bee) lays eggs on a horse's legs in the late summer. When the horse licks his legs, the warmth and moisture cause the larvae to hatch and they are ingested. They travel to the stomach, where they attach to the lining and live until spring, when the greatly enlarged larvae pass out with the feces, pupate in the ground, and hatch into bot flies in the late summer or early fall. The bot fly then continues the cycle. Two ways to break this cycle are to deworm for bots (see* **Deworming***, p. 44) and to regularly remove bot eggs from the horse.*

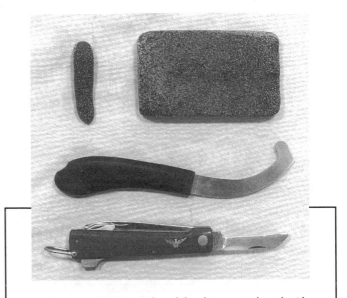

YOU WILL NEED: bot blocks *(top)*, bot knife *(middle)*, pocketknife with blunt safety tip *(bottom)*.

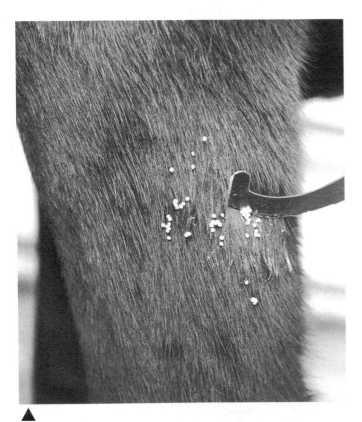

▲
BOT KNIFE
A bot knife has serrated, not sharp, edges and a specially shaped tip that is designed to be safe, yet allow you to get into small nooks and crannies. These bot eggs on this horse's foreleg are easily removed with a simple, scraping motion. Perform this somewhere the horse does not eat; otherwise the horse might ingest the eggs you scrape off.

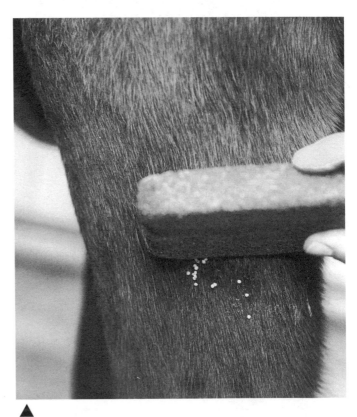

▲
BOT BLOCK
Another way to remove bot eggs is with a bot block, which is a rough, porous stone that rubs the eggs off the hair. As it does, however, the pores of the block fill up with hair and dirt and the edges become rounded, so the block becomes less effective.

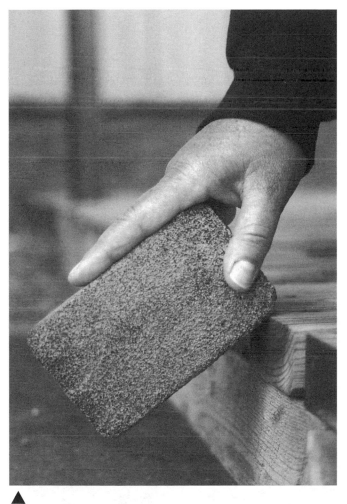

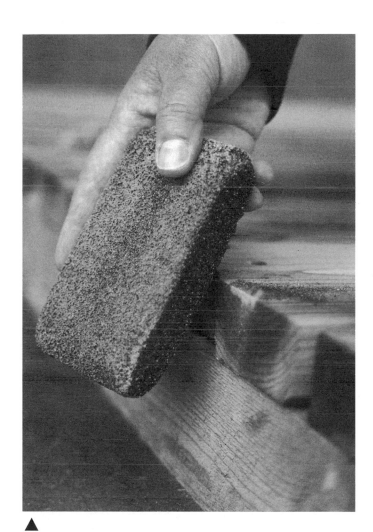

▲
SHARPENING THE BOT BLOCK
To sharpen the block, run it across a sharp edge, such as a board.

▲
SHARPENED BOT BLOCK
Sharpening the bot block cleans the edge of the block, and it will be ready to use again. Note the pile of tiny cinders on the board.

APPLYING FLY SPRAY

Even if you are conscientious about cleaning your horse's stall or pen and you are a good manure manager and you keep the area around the barn dry and free of tall grass and weeds, you probably will still have stable flies during certain months of the summer. At some time or another, you will have to apply fly repellent to your horse. There are certain places that flies are most likely to land on your horse, so that's where you should concentrate your efforts.

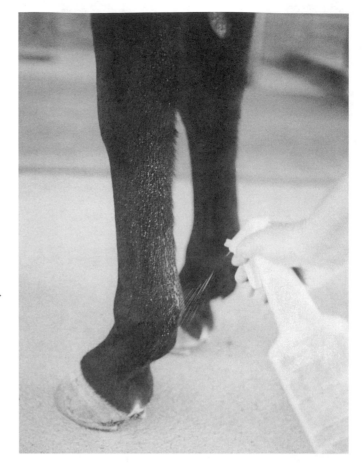

SPRAY THE LOWER LEGS ▶

One of the most important places to apply fly spray is to the lower legs, especially along the back of the horse's legs all the way down to the coronary band. Be sure to get the fetlock and pastern areas as well. This is where a lot of flies land, causing foot stomping. Constant stomping is not only stressful to the horse's limbs but it can be responsible for loose and shifting shoes as well.

SPRAY THE NECK AND CHEST ▶

Another area that attracts gnats and blood-sucking flies is the junction of the horse's neck and chest where the hair tends to whorl and crease and expose bare spots. The chin and jaw are vulnerable spots, too.

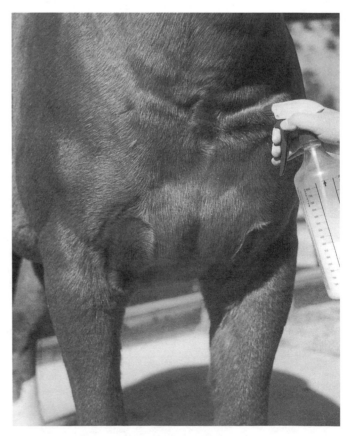

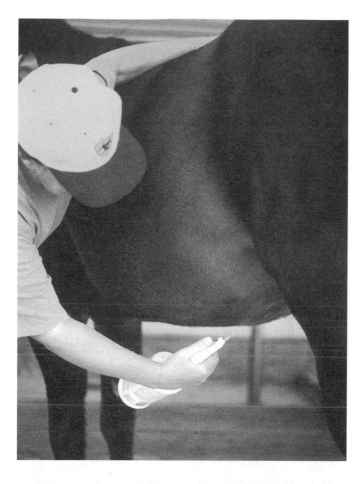

◄ SPRAY THE ABDOMEN

On the horse's abdomen, just in front of the sheath or udder, there is another lightly haired patch of skin where flies like to feast. Pastured horses that aren't sprayed often have crusty scabs here. Use safe handling techniques to keep the horse from moving into or away from you as you spray. Do not spray fly spray directly onto the sheath or udder unless you know for certain that it is a formula that is designed specifically for bare, sensitive skin.

◄ SENSITIVE AREAS

For sensitive areas such as the face, ears, and sheath or udder, you might want to use a fly repellent cream that you apply with a soft cloth or an old terry loop sock turned inside out.

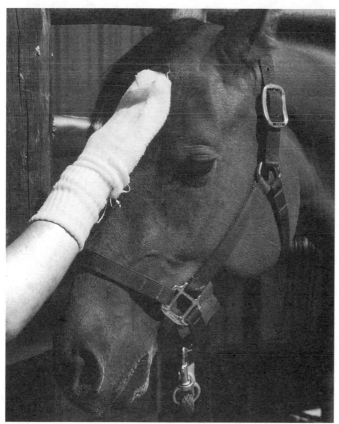

PUTTING ON A FLY MASK

Flies are attracted to the moisture around a horse's eyes, where the flies often cause an inflammation of the conjunctiva, the white membrane that lines the eyelid. The inflammation, called conjunctivitis, causes the lining to become red. The bacteria-laden secretions around the eyes attract more flies and perpetuate the cycle, until the condition can become sight-threatening.

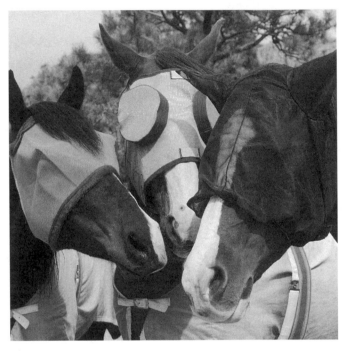

▲
FLY MASKS
Because the use of fly repellents around the sensitive areas of the face is not recommended, fly masks are often used. Most fly masks also minimize the effect of bright sunlight on the horse's eyes.

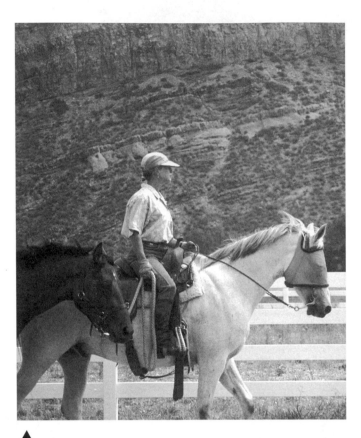

▲
FLY MASKS FOR RIDING
Pasture horses are prime candidates for fly masks, but since horses can see quite well out of most of the fly masks on the market today, fly masks are used for riding as well.

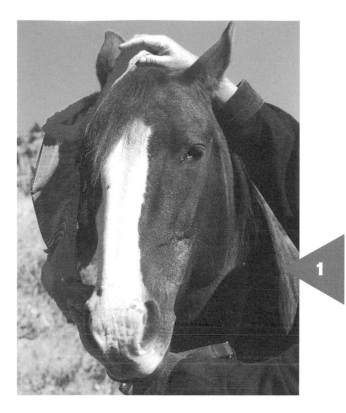

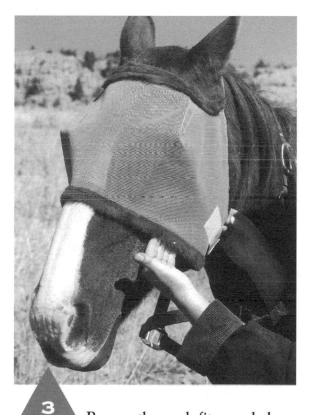 Remove the halter from the horse's head and buckle it around his neck. Bring the fly mask to the off side, such as you would to bridle a horse. Slip the crown piece over the horse's off ear. Move the fly mask over the horse's eyes and bring the crownpiece over the near ear. Be sure the fly mask is the correct size for the horse. The peaked areas should be directly over the horse's eyes.

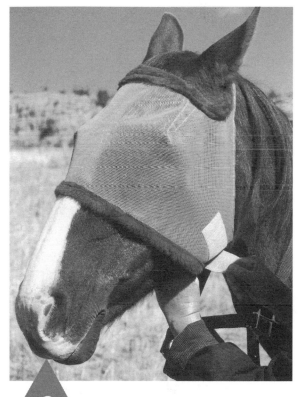

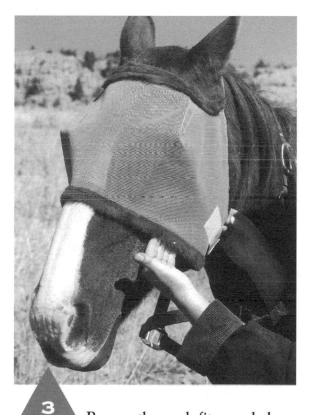

2 Fasten the throatlatch. If the fastener is a hook-and-loop closure, be sure your horse is accustomed to that peculiar sound when it is pulled apart because otherwise it could cause your horse to spook.

3 Be sure the mask fits snugly because you don't want flies to be able to crawl into the mask. If they did, they would be trapped inside the mask and would be very bothersome for your horse. *This mask is too loose.*

Measuring a Horse

MEASURING HEIGHT

Keeping a record of your young horse's height as he grows is very interesting. In some cases, you will need to know your horse's official height for registration or show purposes.

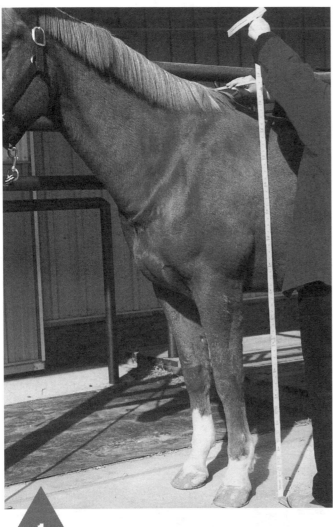

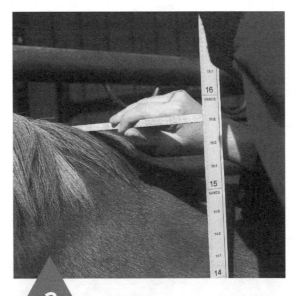

1 Be sure your horse is standing with weight on all four feet and with his legs set squarely under his body, that is, not set out in front of or behind his body exaggeratedly. He should be standing on a flat, level surface, such as on concrete or a rubber mat. Hold the measuring tape vertically and taut in your left hand. Hold a stick on the highest point of your horse's withers with your right hand.

2 Hold the stick horizontal. Take the reading where the bottom of the stick meets the measuring tape. This horse is 15•3 hands tall. A hand equals 4 inches, so this horse is 63 inches tall. 15 hands x 4 inches per hand = 60 inches + 3 inches = 63 inches.

MEASURING WEIGHT

You need to know your horse's weight for routine deworming, other medication dosage, ration formulation, and other uses. Specially calibrated equine weight tapes, when used correctly, will give quite accurate estimates of a horse's weight.

CALCULATING POUNDS

IF YOU DON'T have a specially calibrated weight tape, you can measure your horse's heart girth with an ordinary measuring tape and use the following table to get an estimate of your horse's weight.

GIRTH IN INCHES	WEIGHT IN POUNDS	GIRTH IN INCHES	WEIGHT IN POUNDS
32	100	66	860
40	200	68	930
45	275	70	1000
50	375	72	1070
55	500	74	1140
60	650	76	1210
62	720	78	1290
64	790	80	1370

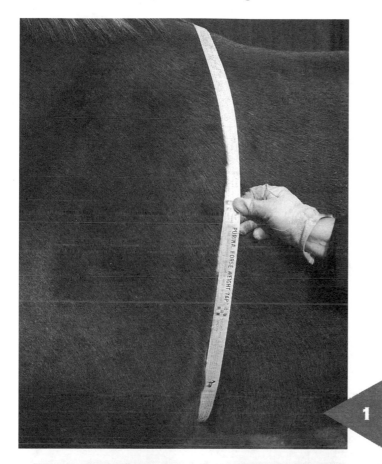

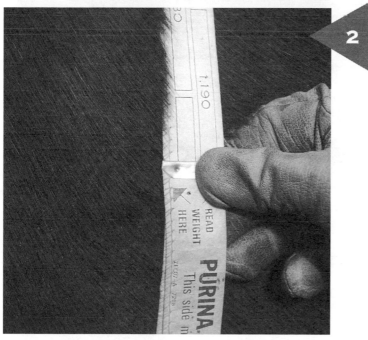

1 With the weight tape, encircle the horse's heart-girth area as shown. Pull the tape up snugly.

2 Read the weight tape as indicated. This horse weighs more than 1190 pounds, but slightly less than 1250, which is the next weight increment on the tape (underneath the thumb). So he could be said to weigh 1240 pounds.

Hoof Care

PICKING OUT THE HOOVES

The cleaner you keep your horse's hooves, the less likely he will be to develop thrush, a decomposition of hoof structures caused by wet, unsanitary footing. Also, if you pick out your horse's hooves daily, you will be more likely to discover problems early.

YOU WILL NEED *(from the left)* a high-quality hoof dressing, hoof sealer, hoof pick.

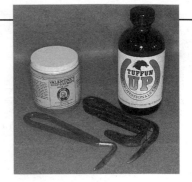

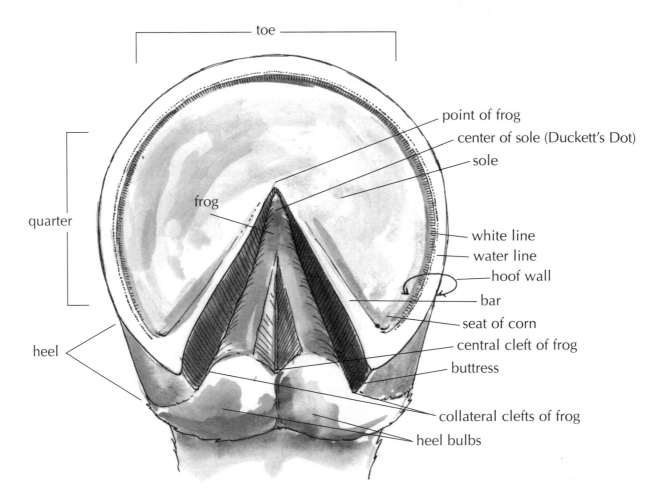

PARTS OF THE HOOF

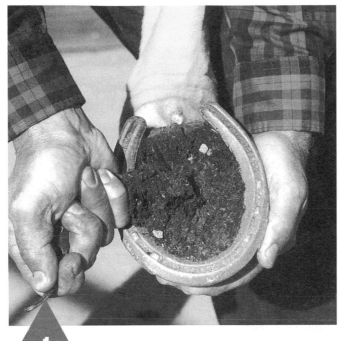

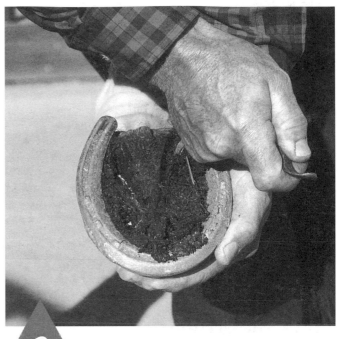

1 Begin by holding the hoof in a comfortable position, with the hoof well supported by one hand. Holding the hoof pick in your other hand, loosen the mud, manure, and bedding by inserting the point of the hoof pick near the bulbs of the heels. Often you will be able to pop off a large disk of mud and manure with this technique.

2 Then make downward swipes with the hoof pick in the clefts of the frog. With practice, you will know exactly where the clefts are even if they are covered over with mud.

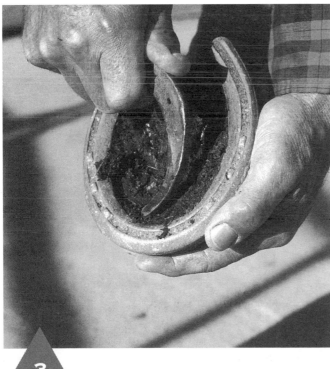

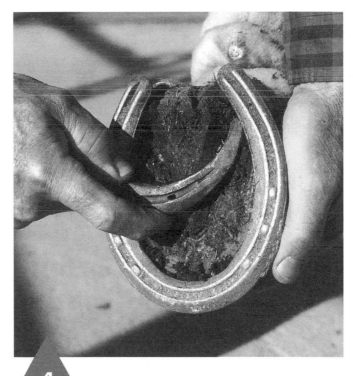

3 Now do a more thorough job of scraping all debris from around the inside edge of the shoe or hoof.

4 Be sure to get any mud or material that has become lodged under the heels of the shoes near the opening of the clefts of the frog.

PERFORMING A HOOF CHECK

After you have picked out your horse's hooves, give them a once-over to spot small problems before they become an emergency.

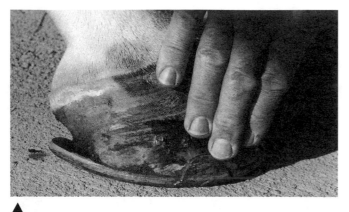

▲
CHECK THE CLINCHES

Run your fingertips over the clinches (the folded-over ends of horseshoe nails on the outside of your horse's hooves) to determine if they are smooth or rough. Feel the clinches right after your horse is freshly shod so you know what your farrier's newly set clinches normally feel like.

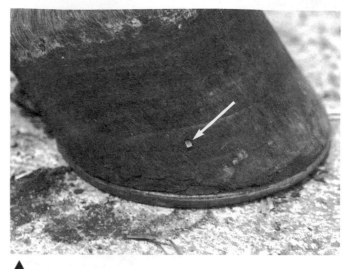

▲
LOOSE CLINCH

A rough clinch could be a loose clinch and indicates the shoe might be shifting on the horse's hoof and might possibly come off. If the clinches are very rough and loose, your farrier will need to come and tighten them or perhaps reshoe your horse. Here is an example of a loose clinch.

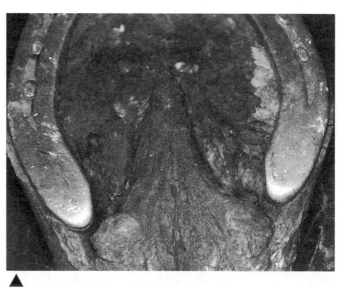

▲
HOOF GROWS OVER SHOE

Look at the bottom of your horse's hooves to see if the hoof has grown over the shoe. Sometimes this will happen rather quickly in wet weather because the hoof tissue expands. But usually this occurs because the horse's shoes have been on too long, longer than 6 or 8 weeks, and the shoes need to be reset. Unlike this photo, you should not see any part of the hoof along the outside edge of the shoe.

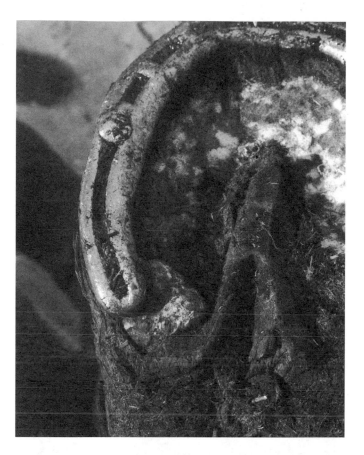

◄ REMOVE FOREIGN OBJECTS

While you are looking at the bottom of your horse's hooves, be sure to note any foreign objects such as this rock, which is caught under the heel of the shoe and is putting pressure on the horse's hoof. Painful bruises often form from such pressure.

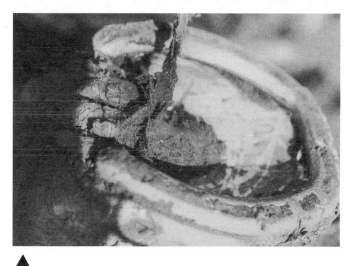

▲ CONDITION OF FROG

This frog has deteriorated and is sloughing; that is, the dead tissue is coming off in layers. Some horses shed their frogs and soles about twice a year, so a ragged frog might just indicate that the horse's frog needs a good trim during the next farrier visit. Or it could mean that there is an unfriendly organism at work destroying the hoof structures. If you are suspicious of the latter, confer with your veterinarian or farrier.

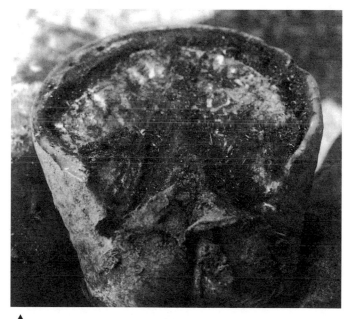

▲ BARE FEET

If your horse is barefoot, he will still need farrier attention. This photo shows a bare hoof that needs a trim. The hoof wall has grown long enough so that if it isn't trimmed, it will begin breaking.

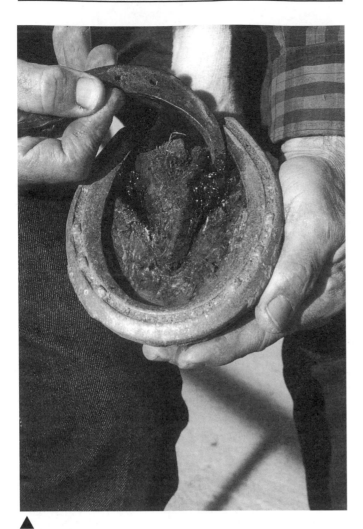

▲

IDENTIFYING THRUSH

Keep your eyes and nose ever vigilant for signs of thrush, a black, foul-smelling decay of hoof tissues. If you see something like this, it is past the time to get your veterinarian or farrier involved. The hoof will have to be pared down to healthy tissue and treated with a special thrush disinfectant.

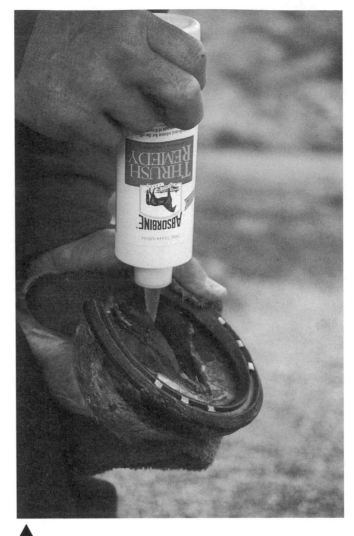

▲

APPLYING THRUSH REMEDIES

Whichever product your farrier recommends, be sure you apply it deep into the clefts of the clean, pared frog.

MAKING A HOME REMEDY FOR THRUSH

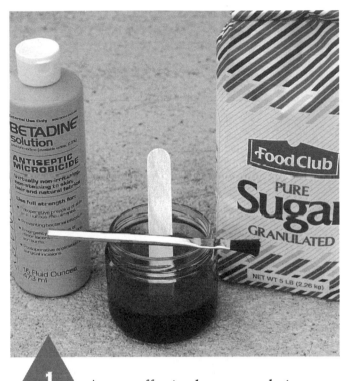

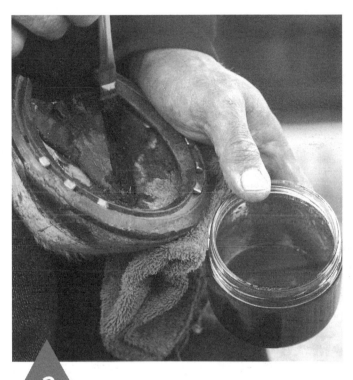

1 A very effective home remedy is sugardyne. Mix ordinary sugar with Betadine 10% Stock Solution until the resulting consistency is like thick honey.

2 Using a small brush, paint the clefts with sugardyne as directed by your farrier or veterinarian.

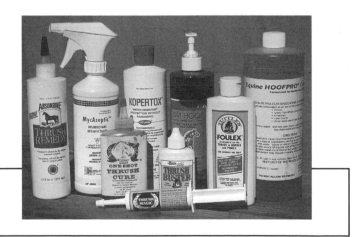

THERE ARE a variety of thrush remedies on the market.

PUTTING ON HOOF SEALER

Hoof sealer is a thin, clear substance that is painted or sprayed onto the hoof wall to help maintain proper hoof moisture. It seals the hoof wall so that precious moisture in the blood within the hoof does not evaporate through the hoof wall. More importantly, it seals excess moisture from entering the hoof through the wall. When a horse is in excessively wet conditions, his hooves can deteriorate quickly.

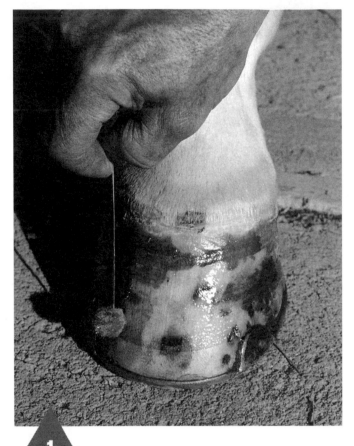

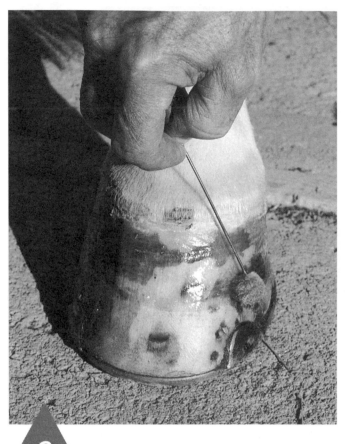

1 To apply a sealer, the hoof must be absolutely clean and dry. With the dauber wet but not dripping with sealer, start just below the coronary band and work back and forth across the hoof wall. Start at the toe and get the center area (called the "toe area") of the hoof, from coronary band to the ground.

2 Then dip the dauber into the sealer and do the same for the inside quarter, then the outside quarter. Let the sealer dry before exposing the hooves to dirt or bedding.

PUTTING ON HOOF DRESSING

A hoof dressing is an oily or greasy substance made from various ingredients, such as petroleum products, fish oil, and lanolin. Natural ingredients are preferred over petroleum products. Hoof dressings do not make the hoof more moist. The best way to get more hoof moisture is to increase the blood flow to the hoof, usually through proper nutrition and exercise.

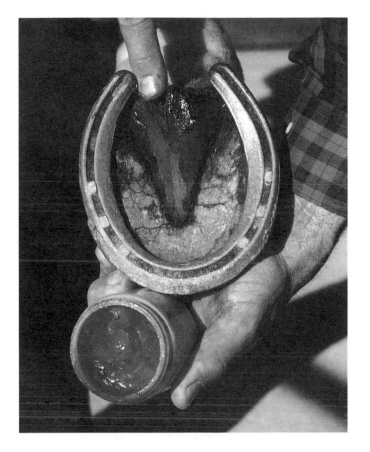

◄ WHEN TO USE HOOF DRESSING

Hoof dressings should not be overused. In fact, there are only a few instances when a hoof dressing is necessary or desirable. When the heels of a horse's hoof have become dry and cracked, they can be softened with a daily application of a dressing, such as this fish oil–based dressing. It should be applied discriminately and rubbed in thoroughly.

PREVENTING LOOSE AND LOST SHOES

To prevent loose and lost shoes, follow these recommendations:

+ Do not pasture shod horses in wet or boggy fields.

+ Do not subject a horse's hooves to repeated wet–dry episodes, such as frequent baths or leg rinsing.

+ Pick out a horse's hooves regularly. Removing manure and mud from a horse's hooves will allow them to dry and remain more durable.

+ Use a knowledgeable and experienced farrier.

+ Keep horses on a regular shoeing program, every 6 to 8 weeks or as your farrier advises.

+ Keep the horse fit and in shape. A well-conditioned horse generally moves in better balance and has less chance of stepping off a shoe due to fatigue.

+ Check the shoes and nail heads regularly for signs of wear or damage.

+ Check the clinches regularly to see if they are loose.

REMOVING A LOOSE SHOE

A loose or bent horseshoe requires immediate attention. A loose shoe can swivel on the hoof, exposing the dislodged horseshoe nails. If a horse steps on these nails, he could puncture his sole. The nails could cut the horse's other leg when he moves. And if a loose shoe is not removed, the horse will likely step on it, ripping the shoe off along with large hunks of hoof wall.

If a loose shoe is forcibly pried off with a screwdriver or yanked off with a claw hammer, large portions of hoof wall may be damaged in the process. In addition, the sole, frog, or heel bulbs could be bruised from the pressure. To avoid further complications, therefore, a loose or bent shoe should be removed properly and the hoof protected until the farrier can replace the shoe.

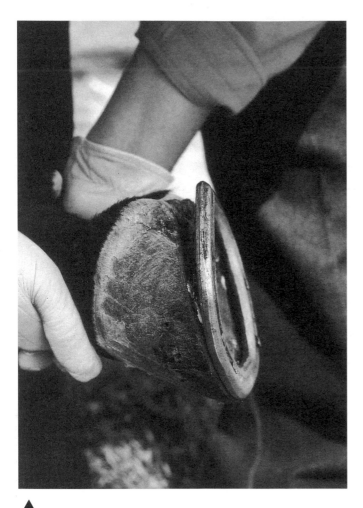

▲
BENT SHOE
The inside branch of this shoe has been stepped on and bent.

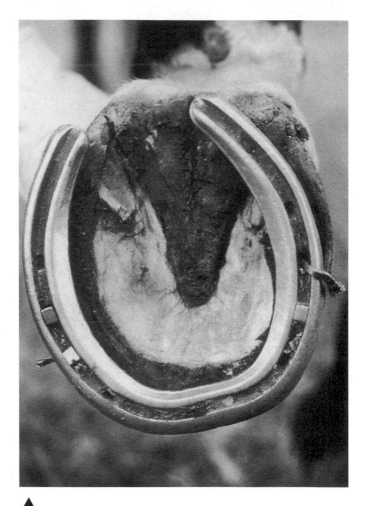

▲
LOOSE SHOE
This shoe has come loose and twisted on the hoof. If not removed, the horse risks injury to the hoof.

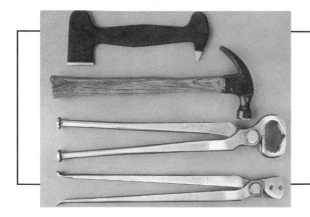

SOME BASIC TOOLS will allow you to remove a shoe safely and easily: *(from top)* clinch cutter, hammer, pull-offs, and crease nail puller.

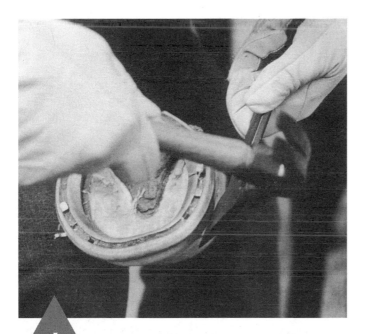

1 To remove a loose shoe, use the chisel end of the clinch cutter and open the clinches by tapping the spine of the clinch cutter with the hammer. (The *clinch* is the end of the nail that has been folded over to form a hook.)

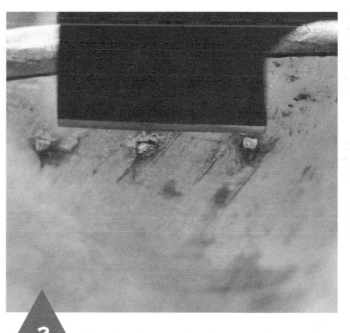

2 The clinches need to be opened up so that the nails can slide straight through the hoof wall when pulled — without taking large hunks of hoof with them.

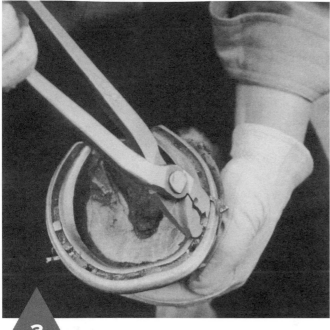

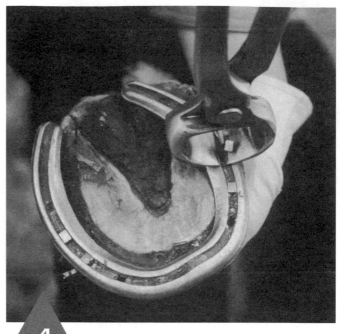

3 If the shoe has a crease on the bottom, you may be able to use the crease nail puller to grab the nail heads and extract each nail individually, allowing the shoe to come off.

4 Nails with protruding heads can be pulled out using the pull-offs.

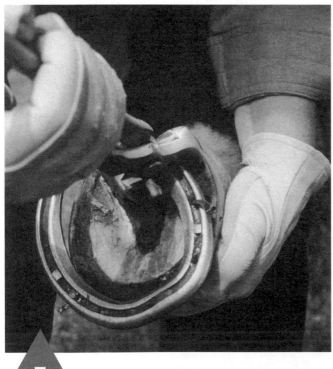

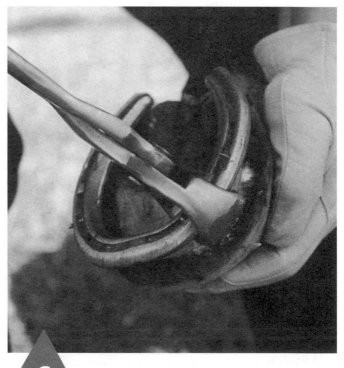

5 If you can't pull the nails out individually, you will have to remove the shoe with the pull-offs. After the clinches have been opened, grab the shoe heel that is most securely attached and pry toward the tip of the frog. Do the same with the other shoe heel.

6 When both heels are loose, grab one side of the shoe at the toe and pry toward the tip of the frog. Repeat around the shoe until it is removed. **NEVER** pry toward the outside of the hoof or you risk ripping big chunks out of the hoof wall. As the nail heads protrude from the loosening of the shoe, you can pull them out individually with the pull-offs.

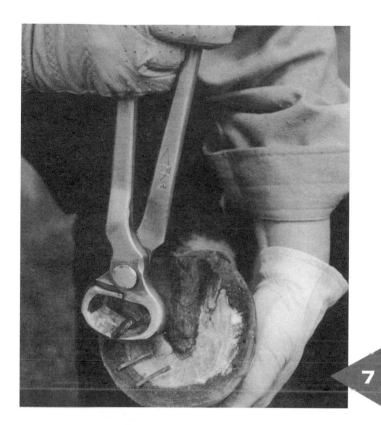

Pull any nails that remain in the hoof. Use the pull-offs to straighten the nail, and pull straight out to avoid damage to the hoof. **7**

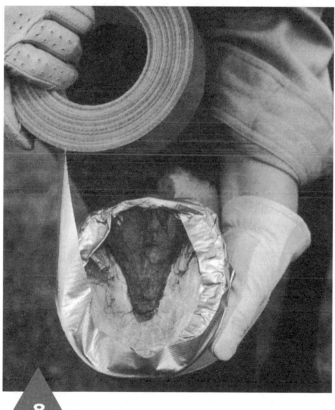

8 Keep the horse confined in an area with soft, dry footing until the shoe can be replaced. To keep the hoof from wearing or chipping until the farrier can replace the shoe, use some sort of hoof protection, such as duct tape.

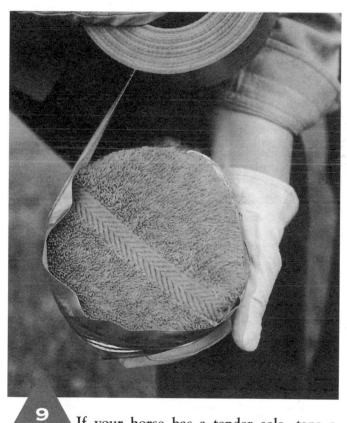

9 If your horse has a tender sole, tape a cloth over the bottom of the hoof with duct tape until the farrier can come to replace the shoe.

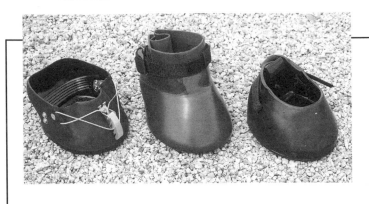

TYPES OF BOOTS

Instead of taping the hoof, you can use a rubber boot to protect the bare hoof until the farrier arrives. There are several styles to choose from. Be sure the boot is the proper size.

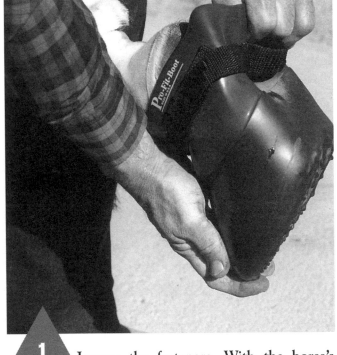

1 Loosen the fasteners. With the horse's lower leg resting across your thighs, use one hand to open the boot and one to guide it on. When you feel the toe of his hoof has arrived at the toe of the boot, you can let him put his foot down, which will secure the boot on his hoof.

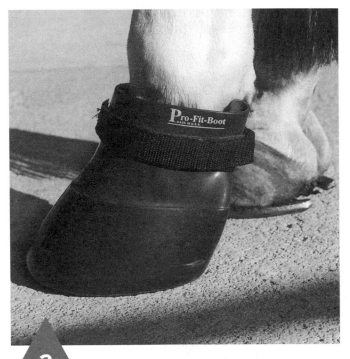

2 Fasten the boot and check to be sure the boot is not rubbing his heels, pastern, or fetlock. This type of boot also functions as a soaking boot if your farrier or vet instructs you to do so for a sole abscess.

Caring for Wounds and Abrasions

PUTTING TOGETHER A FIRST AID KIT

Assemble a first aid kit and keep all the items together for emergencies (see p. 5). Make sure you have your veterinarian's phone number in an easy-to-find place near all of your phones. The purpose of a first aid kit is to provide you with the tools and supplies you need to give immediate care to your horse. Keep the kit clean, easily accessible, and at room temperature. You won't want to have to run around and gather everything and then wash or disinfect things before you can use them. The use of many of the items in this kit will be described in detail in other skills.

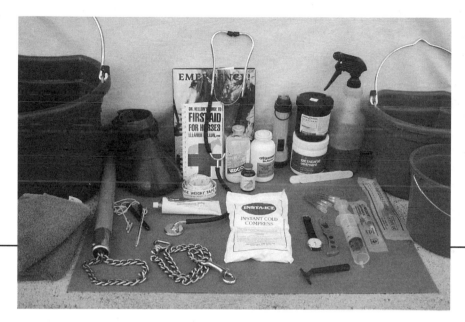

KEEP GOOD FIRST AID BOOKS near your kit. Become very familiar with first aid procedures from these books BEFORE an emergency. In addition to a good selection of clean towels and pails, have the following on hand (from in front of the books, clockwise):

- ✦ Stethoscope
- ✦ Liquid antibiotics (refrigerate)
- ✦ Epinephrine (antidote for anaphylactic shock; refrigerate)
- ✦ Phenylbutazone (anti-inflammatory to relieve pain and swelling; tablets or paste)
- ✦ Flashlight and fresh batteries
- ✦ Two types of wound ointments (Betadine and nitrofurazone)
- ✦ Wooden sticks for removing and spreading ointment
- ✦ Betadine solution in a spray bottle

- ✦ Disposable syringes and needles
- ✦ Pocketknife
- ✦ Watch
- ✦ Disposable razor
- ✦ Instant cold compress
- ✦ Chain
- ✦ Twitch
- ✦ Thermometer
- ✦ Protective boot
- ✦ Weight and height tape
- ✦ Lubricating jelly

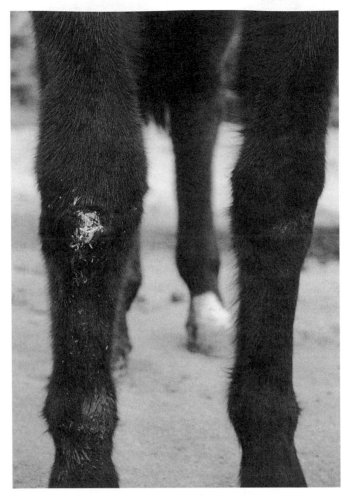

▲

PUNCTURE WOUND

This is a wound on a young horse's knee. Because there is very little muscle tissue in this area, the wound could have penetrated the joint capsule, which would be cause for alarm because of the possibility of joint infection. A puncture wound is a serious wound and should be treated by your veterinarian.

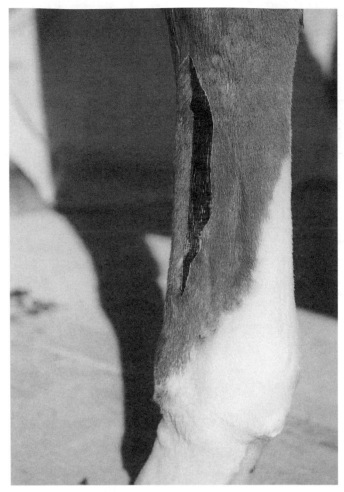

▲

ABRASION OR LACERATION?

The lower limb is the most common site for a wound. If just hair and a few layers of skin are missing, the wound is an abrasion, which is basically a scrape. If the skin has become separated or cut, the wound is a laceration. Some lacerations heal fine without stitching; others require suturing.

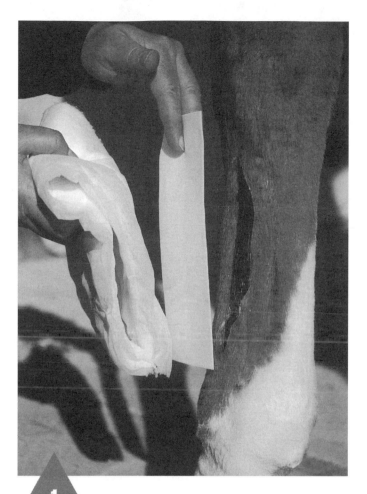

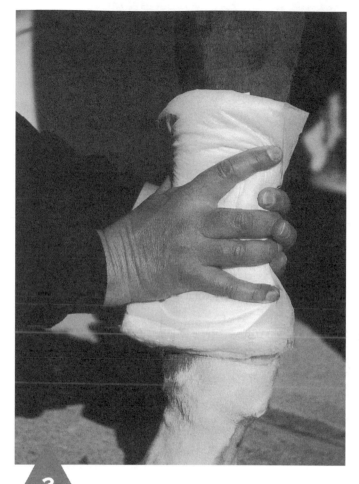

1 If the wound is bleeding heavily, your first concern is to stop the bleeding. You can do this in several ways. One is by applying a pressure bandage until the veterinarian arrives. (See **Bandaging a Wound, p. 79.**) You would only do that if the wound was bleeding very heavily and you knew the veterinarian would be there very soon. Normally, you would not want to bandage a wound that has not been cleaned and clipped first. If the wound is bleeding and you are going to prepare and dress it yourself, first stop the bleeding this way: Place a nonstick gauze square (one with a special plastic coating) over the bleeding area and cover it with a thick layer of cotton bandaging material. The nonstick pad is necessary because once you stop the bleeding and you want to remove the pad to clean and clip the wound, a nonstick pad comes right off. A regular gauze pad will tear away the clot that has formed and the bleeding will begin again.

2 Press firmly on the area that is bleeding. Sometimes this is all that is necessary. You can also apply a crepe bandage with tension over the cotton batting. Such a wrap should only be left on temporarily to stop the bleeding.

USING GAUZE PADS

When dressing a wound after heavy bleeding has stopped, apply a regular, woven gauze pad. The gauze pad absorbs the wound secretions, lifts them, and stores them away from the wound surface. When the bandage is removed and the gauze pad is peeled off, it naturally removes the wound debris. Once a wound begins closing and you don't want to disturb the healing wound surface, you can start using a nonstick pad. This shift in wound dressings usually takes place from 3 to 14 days after injury.

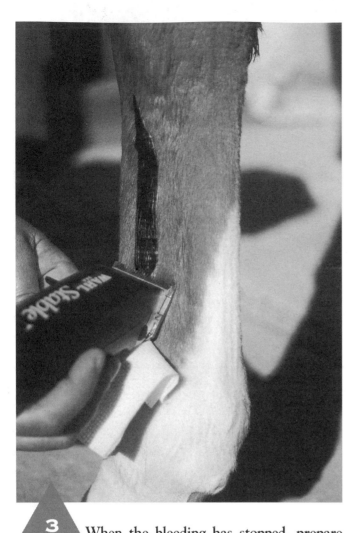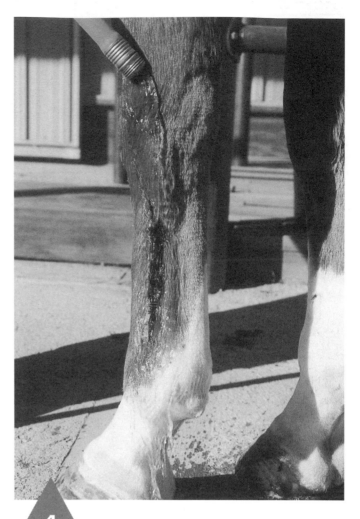

3 When the bleeding has stopped, prepare the wound for permanent bandaging. Clip the hair from the edges of the wound. Clean, shaved skin will have an easier time healing because it is less prone to harboring bacteria and debris. A clean wound edge will knit together more smoothly and with less chance of a scar than will ragged, hairy edges. To keep the hair clippings from falling into the wound itself, hold a square of damp gauze underneath the clipper blades. That will act like a hair magnet as you clip upward, against the direction of hair growth. Use a #30 or #40 (surgical) blade on your clippers. You might also be able to do a good job of shaving off the hair with a disposable razor.

4 If the wound area is very dirty, thoroughly flush the clipped wound site with cold water. Hold the hose above the wound and let the cold water run over the wound. The water should be coming out in a heavy trickle, not with force. High pressure could send debris into the wound or could injure tissues further, causing bleeding to start again. Cold water should be used, not warm. Cold water diminishes bleeding by causing capillaries to contract. Cold also has a soothing, anti-inflammatory effect on the traumatized tissues. Usually 3 to 5 minutes of cold flushing suffices. Longer hosing results in waterlogged tissues that have a more difficult time healing.

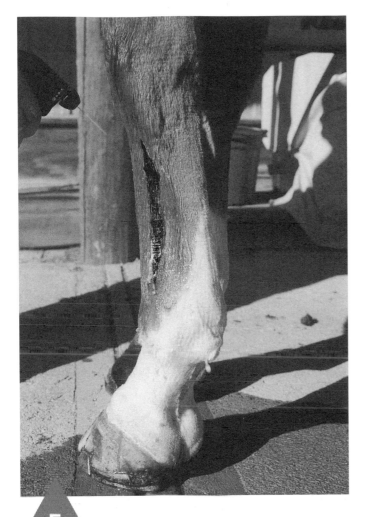

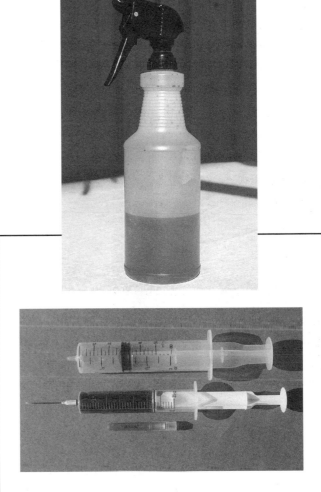

5 The wound should be disinfected by spraying with a wound wash such as povidone iodine saline solution. The recipe and instructions follow in the next skill.

APPLICATION OF WOUND WASH

The wound wash can be applied with a 16-oz. spray bottle or a 35 or 60 cc syringe outfitted with an 18-gauge needle. Both deliver a squirt with a pressure of about 7 psi (pounds/square inch). Pressures lower than 7 don't do a good job of removing all debris.

MAKING A WOUND WASH

For flushing wounds, make an appropriate wound wash such as povidone iodine saline solution. If you need a substantial amount of wound wash to treat a large wound over a long period of time, follow the directions for making a gallon. Otherwise, refer to the chart for the amounts necessary to make a quart.

WOUND WASH		
	TO MAKE A GALLON	TO MAKE A QUART
Distilled water	1 gallon	1 quart
Table salt	2.4 tbsp. (36 g)	1.8 tsp. (9 g)
Povidone iodine	1.6 tsp. (8 ml)	.4 tsp. (2 ml)

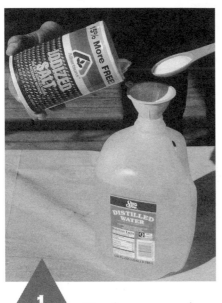

1 Purchase or make saline solution. To make: Remove a bit of water from a gallon jug of distilled water. Add 2½ tablespoons of table salt. Shake to dissolve and distribute the salt throughout the water.

HANDY CONVERSIONS (APPROXIMATIONS)

30 grams	=	1 ounce
2 tablespoons	=	1 ounce
30 ml	=	1 fluid ounce
5 ml	=	1 teaspoon
15 ml	=	1 tablespoon
30 ml	=	2 tablespoons
3 teaspoons	=	1 tablespoon

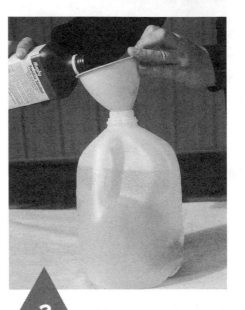

2 Add some povidone iodine solution to the saline solution you have just made. *Do not* use tincture of iodine; it is too harsh. *Do not* use an iodine "scrub," which is an iodine solution with soap in it, because the soap can interfere with wound healing. *Povidone iodine* (the trade name is Betadine) is tamed iodine that has already been diluted to a 10% solution. You will be diluting it even further. Research has found that a certain very weak concentration of povidone iodine is best for preventing bacterial infection without being so strong as to damage tender tissues as they heal. The proportions listed here are based on that research. To the gallon of saline solution, add a scant 2 teaspoons (about 8 ml) of povidone iodine solution. The resulting solution should look like weak tea. This solution is suitable for flushing and disinfecting wounds.

BANDAGING A WOUND

A properly applied wound bandage serves many functions. It protects the wound from contamination by dirt, bedding, and airborne particles; it exerts an appropriate amount of pressure and support which holds the wound edges in an advantageous position for healing and prevents tissue swelling; it keeps the wound site warm, prevents the wound from drying out, and provides protection from inevitable bumps to the vulnerable tissues.

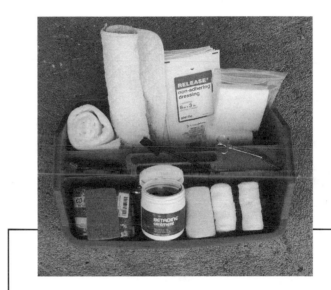

YOUR WOUND BANDAGING KIT can be assembled in a handy tote that can be carried to the horse's side: *(top row from left)* 14" x 30" cotton batting, 12" x 30" cotton leg quilt, 8" x 3" sterile nonstick dressings, 4" x 4" gauze squares in plastic bag; (middle row) bandage cutting knife, small brush, bandage scissors; (bottom row) 4" x 5 yards stretchable, conforming crepe bandage, Betadine ointment, 4" x 5 yards elastic conforming adhesive tape, rolls of 4" x 3 yards conforming, clinging gauze.

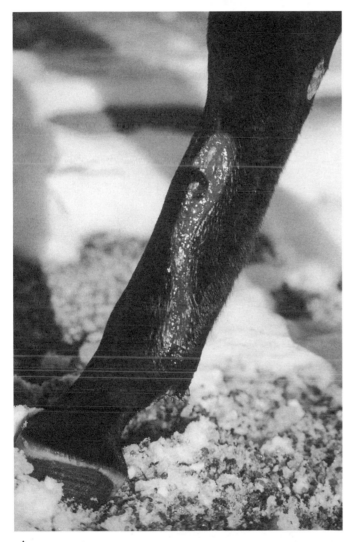

▲
FRESH WOUND
This wound on the inside of the right hind leg is only hours old. The bleeding stopped on its own. It has not been cleaned or clipped. Some of the ragged skin flaps will have to be trimmed away.

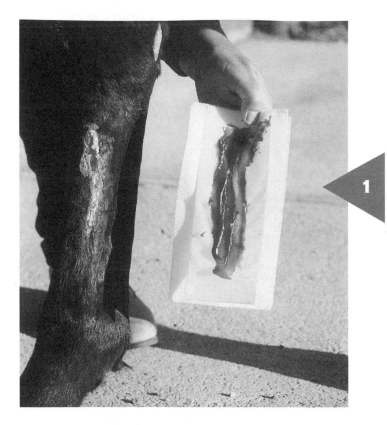

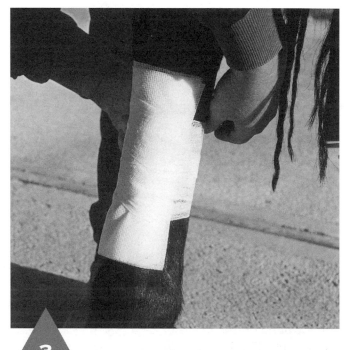

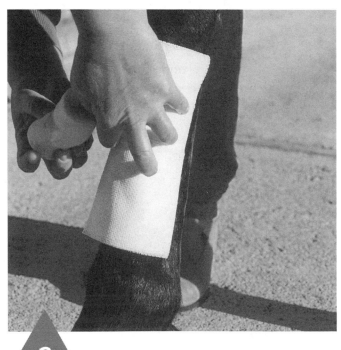

1 The edges of the same wound, several weeks old, have already started to pull together. The wound area was cleaned with wound wash, using a spray bottle or syringe as previously described. This method removes debris without disturbing the healing. Betadine ointment is spread on the nonstick pad (see "Using Gauze Pads," p. 75) in a pattern corresponding to the size and shape of the wound. Triple antibiotic ointment is also very good to use. Also with the nonstick pad are three 4" x 4" gauze squares that have been opened so they are now 4" x 8". These gauze squares will provide some cushioning over the wound.

2 The nonstick pad with ointment and the opened gauze squares are laid over the wound and held in place while a 4" roll of conforming, clinging gauze is opened.

3 The gauze is wrapped around the dressing with moderate tension, just enough to hold the dressing in place. Too loose and the dressing will slip inside the bandage. Too tight and it can cause the horse to chew at the bandage. It could also result in pressure damage to the horse's tendons or skin.

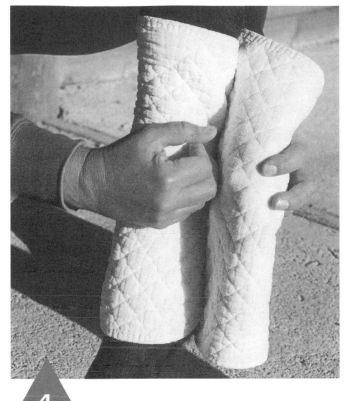

▶ **4** Wrap either some cotton batting or a cotton leg quilt snugly around the cannon.

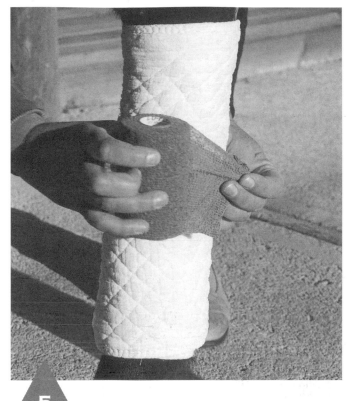

▶ **5** While holding it in place, start a roll of elastic conforming crepe bandage.

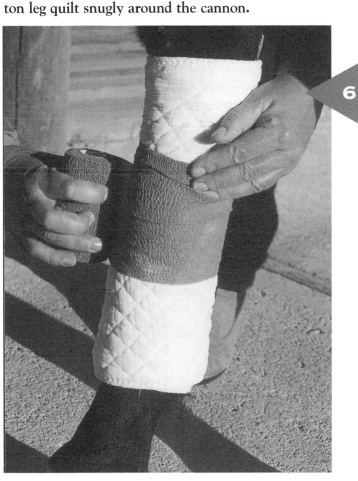

◀ **6** Wrap the bandage around the padding with firm, even pressure. There is less chance of pressure discomfort or problems now that there are several thick layers of padding on the limb. Wrap down toward the bottom of the bandage first but leave ½" of padding emerging from the bottom of the bandage. This is more comfortable for the horse because you won't inadvertently end up with a sharp edge of pressure as you would if the elastic tape were the edge of the bandage.

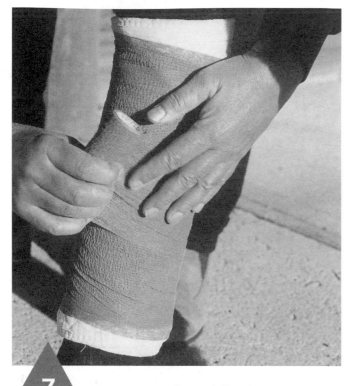

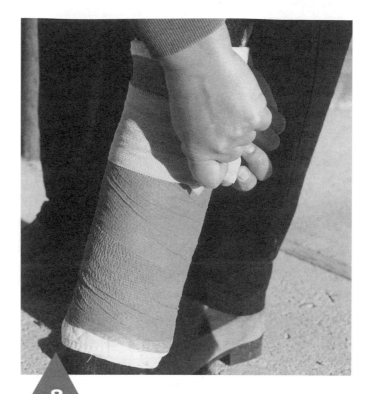

7 Wrap up past the middle where you started, up to the top, leaving some padding exposed. Then wrap down to the middle where you began. You should be about out of crepe bandaging material.

8 Try to plan so that you end somewhere near the center. Cut a 10" piece of elastic conforming adhesive tape and place it securely over the end of the crepe bandage.

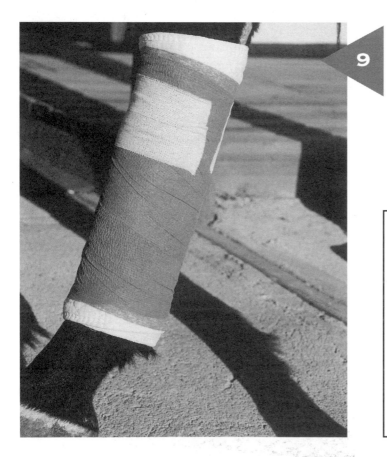

9 Here is the finished bandage. Note: The ends of the adhesive tape do not meet. This is desirable. A single piece of elastic tape in an incomplete ring has little chance of causing a pressure problem.

HOW LONG SHOULD A BANDAGE STAY ON?

When a wound is fresh, the bandage can be changed every day for 2 or 3 days because there might be large amounts of wound discharge and possible sloughing of dead tissue. After that, a bandage can stay on for 2 or 3 days. When the wound starts drying up quite well (after 4 or 5 weeks), it is possible to leave a bandage on for 4 or 5 days at a time.

REMOVING A BANDAGE

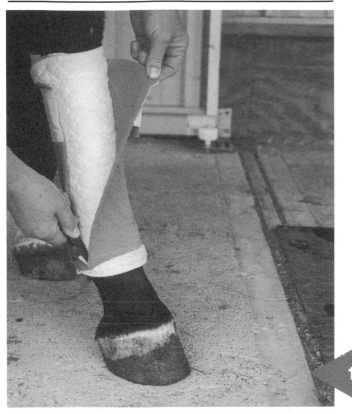

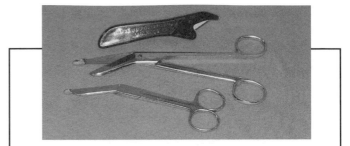

YOU CAN REMOVE a bandage using special blunt-ended bandage scissors or using a special bandage-cutting knife.

1 Using a handy bandage-cutting knife, you can easily slit the outer layer of bandage material in one quick move.

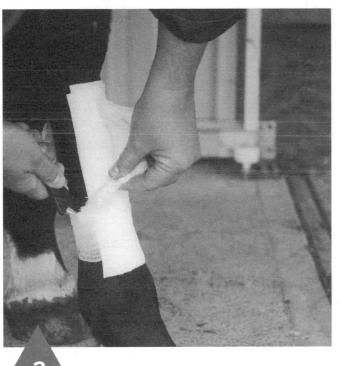

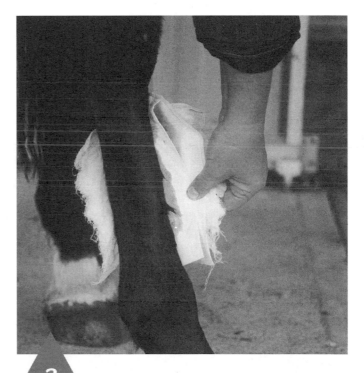

2 The same technique is used on the gauze that was rolled over the wound dressing, but it takes a little more time and patience.

3 When removing the dressing, sometimes some of the hair or wound secretions can cause even a non-stick pad to adhere slightly. It is best to remove the dressing with one quick pull. If you try to peel it off slowly, the horse is liable to jerk his foot away or even kick.

APPLYING
A LIGHT BANDAGE

After a wound has dried up and the edges have come together fairly well, it is no longer necessary to use thick padding and pressure to hold the wound together and protect it.

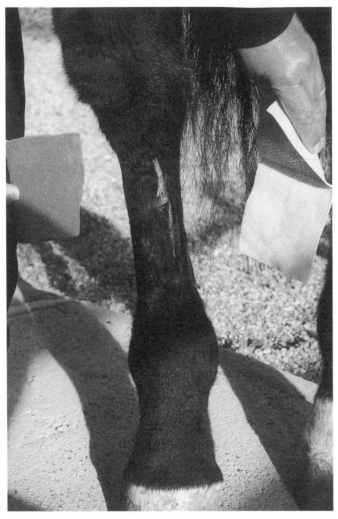

▲
TOUGHENING UP A WOUND SITE

This shows the same wound as in the previous skills, but seven weeks after injury. It is still a good idea to provide some protection from cold air, dirt, and possible bumps. After a limb has been bandaged for several weeks, the tissue around the wound has become somewhat vulnerable and bandage-dependent. To help a wound site get used to the outside world once again, to toughen it up slowly, you can apply a light bandage. This consists of a dry gauze pad, held in place by crepe bandage.

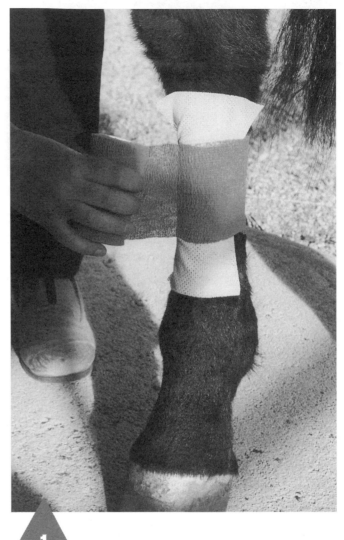

1 Wrap the crepe around the dry gauze dressing. Although it took an entire roll of crepe bandage for a standard wound bandage, you will be able to make three light bandages with one roll.

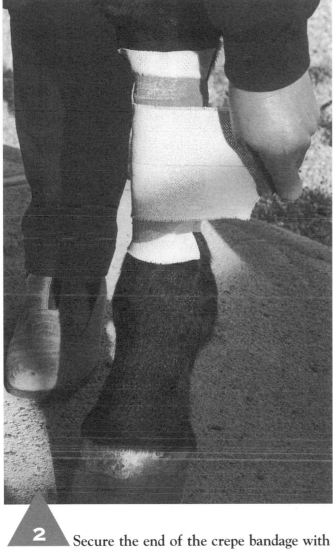

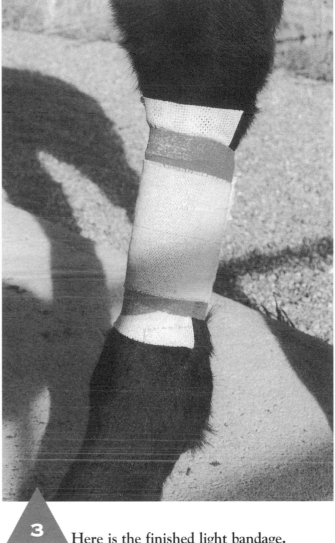

2 Secure the end of the crepe bandage with elastic adhesive tape.

3 Here is the finished light bandage.

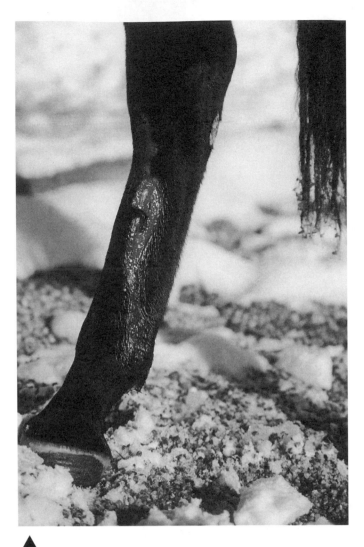

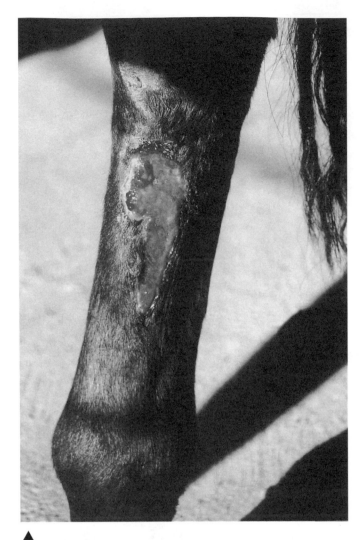

▲
A FRESH WOUND
This is a fresh wound, untrimmed, unclipped, unwashed. It is several hours old.

▲
WEEK ONE
The same wound one week later, showing the bed of granulation tissue that has spanned the open space and filled in the wound.

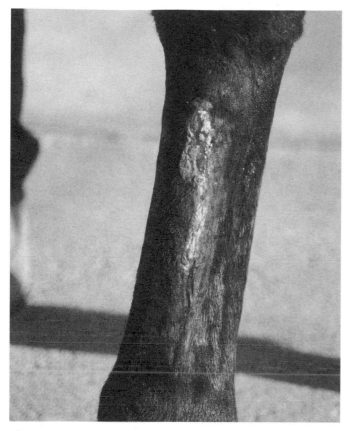

▲
Week Four
Four weeks after injury, the wound has greatly diminished in size and has a good network of protective scabs.

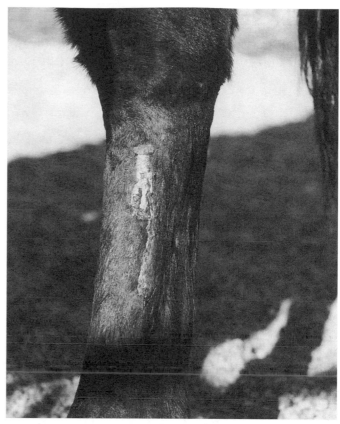

▲
Week Seven
The full bandage was still in use until week seven. At week seven, the light bandage was used for one week.

◄ ## Week Eight
Eight weeks after injury, the light bandage was no longer needed. The wound was rubbed with a lanolin ointment several times a week to keep it soft and pliable.

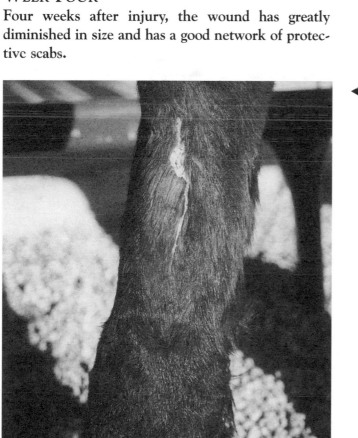

PUTTING ON A MUZZLE

Sometimes it is necessary to put a muzzle on a horse to keep him from chewing a bandage or a healing wound.

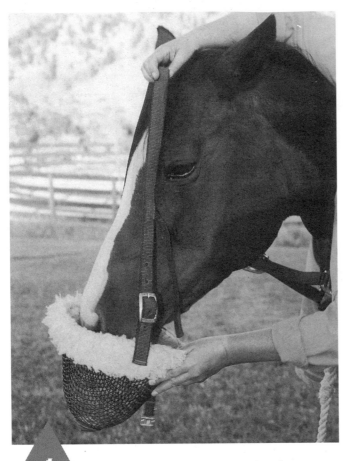

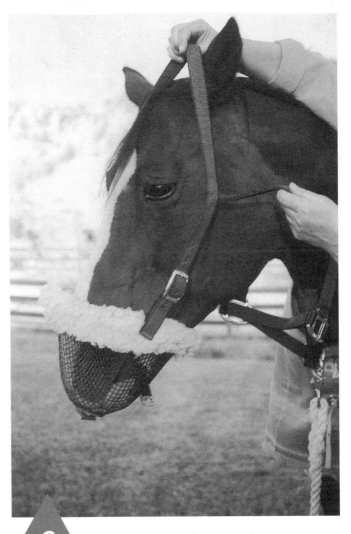

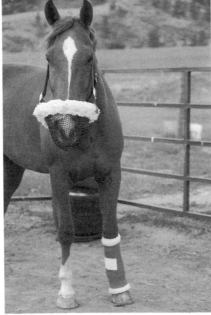

1 Suspend the crownpiece of the muzzle in your right hand and position the muzzle with your left hand.

2 Bring your right hand between the horse's ears just as you do when you are bridling. Bring the basket into position with your left hand, taking care not to bump the horse's eyes. If your horse does not like being muzzled, you can place one or two large wafers in the basket beforehand to give him reason to form a positive association with the muzzle.

◀ MUZZLED HORSE
A muzzled horse will be unable to chew on a bandage or a healing wound.

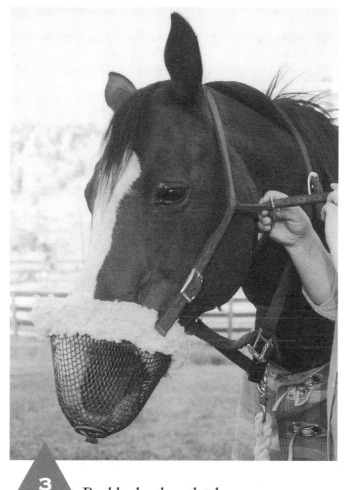

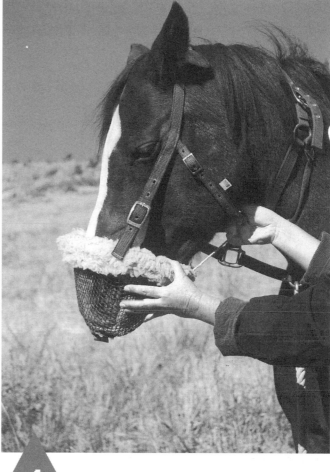

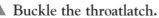
▲ **3** Buckle the throatlatch.

▲ **4** If you find your horse flips the muzzle off over the front of his nose, tie a string from the throatlatch to the rear of the muzzle to prevent this.

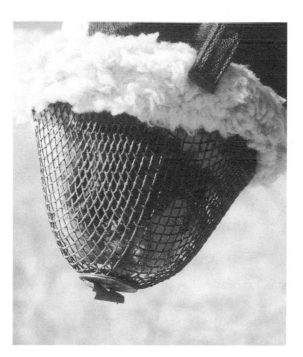

◀ **ADJUST THE HEAD STALL**
The head stall of this muzzle is adjusted too short and has cramped the horse's nose. The head stall should be loosened a hole or two.

USES FOR A MUZZLE

Another use is the case of a broodmare who is turned out on pasture with her foal. Pasture turnout is often more for the foal's benefit because mares can get too fat from the lush feed. The mare wears a muzzle when the pasture is very lush and it slows down or stops her eating while she is out on pasture.

Administering an Intramuscular Injection

Sometime your veterinarian might ask you to give your horse antibiotic injections for several days to help treat an illness or prevent infection in a wound. Confer with your veterinarian as to the type and amount of antibiotics to administer, and know your horse's weight. The following instructions are to familiarize you with the procedure.

NEEDLE SIZE

An 18-gauge needle 1.5" long (also called 18 x 1½) is the preferred needle size for administering an intramuscular injection of liquid antibiotic to a horse. As the numbers get larger, the size of the needle gets smaller. So, a 20-gauge needle is smaller than 18 gauge and although such a needle would insert easily, it is too thin to dispense a thick liquid. The preferred length is 1½" to get the liquid where it needs to go, deep into the muscle tissue. A shorter needle would more likely deposit the antibiotic too superficially under the skin. A longer needle would present dangerous risks of contacting bone or joint structures.

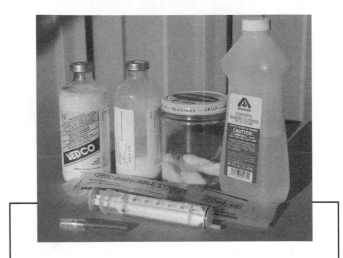

YOU WILL NEED (from left) liquid antibiotic (full bottle and partially used bottle), cotton swabs soaked in alcohol in jar with tight-fitting lid, isopropyl alcohol, disposable sterile syringes, and needles.

FILLING A SYRINGE WITH ANTIBIOTICS

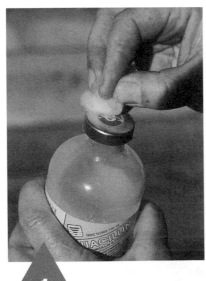

1 Wipe the top of the antibiotic bottle with an alcohol-soaked cotton swab. You can use either isopropyl or ethyl alcohol.

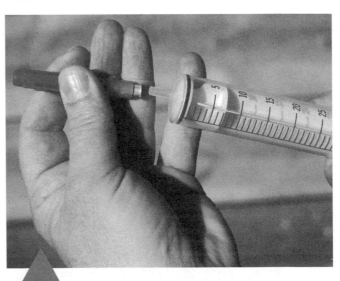

2 With the protective cap still on the needle, attach an 18-gauge 1.5" needle to a sterile 35 cc syringe. Note whether you are using a needle with a slip-on hub or a screw-on hub. The syringe must be of corresponding type.

90

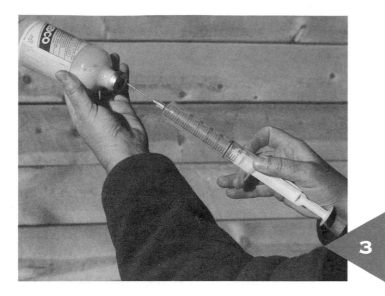

3 Remove the protective cap from the needle. Pull the syringe's plunger out to about the 30 cc mark.

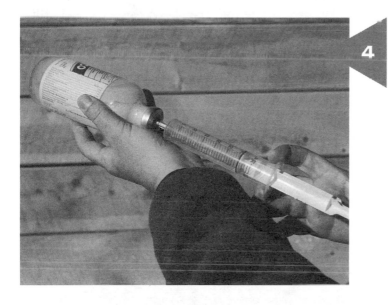

4 Insert the needle into the rubber bottle top. Angle the bottle so that the tip of the needle is in the air space above the liquid. Depress the plunger to add air to the bottle. This will make it easier to draw out the liquid. Note: If you insert the air into the liquid itself, you will create bubbles in the liquid that can make filling the syringe more difficult and will make dispensing the bubbly liquid uneven and possibly dangerous.

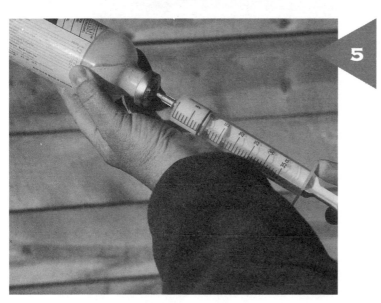

5 Now position the needle tip so that it is in the liquid and begin drawing back on the plunger until you get the required dose, often 20 or 30 cc. Note: You will have to exert more effort pulling back on the plunger when the bottle is almost empty than you did when the bottle was full. Put the protective cap back on the needle until you are ready to administer the injection. You can hold the barrel of the syringe in your hands or under your armpit to bring the temperature of the refrigerated antibiotic closer to body temperature before administering.

INTRAMUSCULAR INJECTION SITES

There are several ways to give an injection: in the vein (intravenous), under the skin (subcutaneous), and in the muscle (intramuscular). Intravenous injections should not be attempted by the horse owner. The risks are too great. Subcutaneous injections are suitable for administering dog vaccines, but they have little application with horses. The third method, intramuscular (IM) injection, is common and appropriate for horse vaccinations and antibiotic administration. Ask your veterinarian to help you administer your first IM injection. The following will help familiarize you with the process.

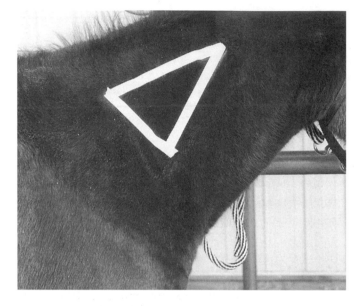

◀ SIDE OF THE NECK

IM injections are given in places of the body where the muscle tissue is thick. The safest and most conventional areas are the side of the neck, the buttocks, and the chest. When a horse is on a long antibiotic regimen, it is necessary to rotate among all six areas (two on each side), so no one spot gets sore. The area inside the triangle on this 2-year-old filly's neck is the most common site for an IM injection.

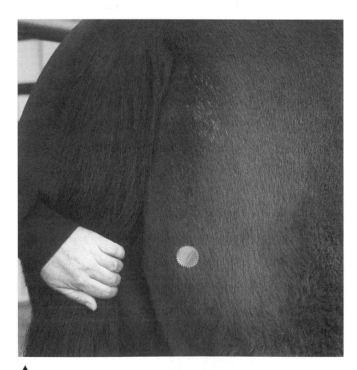

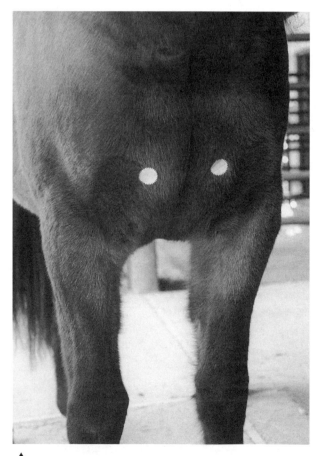

▲
BUTTOCKS
The area of the buttocks approximately indicated by this dot is another safe IM injection site.

▲
CHEST
The two dots on the chest of this filly show yet another IM injection site.

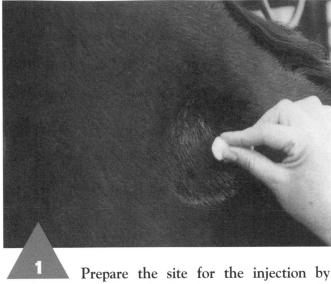

1 Prepare the site for the injection by removing loose hair and debris by grooming or washing and thoroughly drying. Then clean the spot with an alcohol swab. In some instances, your veterinarian might instruct you to clip the injection site.

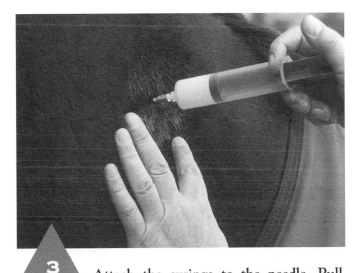

2 Remove the cap from the needle on the filled syringe. Remove any air bubbles by tapping the upright syringe until the air bubbles rise to the needle hub. Slowly depress the plunger to push the air out of the needle. Take the needle off the syringe. Holding the needle perpendicular to the muscle tissue, insert the needle all the way into the muscle with one quick motion.

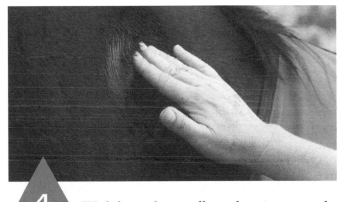

3 Attach the syringe to the needle. Pull back the plunger just a bit (*aspirate*) to see if any blood appears in the white liquid. If you see blood enter the syringe, it means a small blood vessel has been crossed. Withdraw the needle about 1/16" and aspirate again, or choose another site. If you target the area correctly, use the correct size needle, and insert the needle perpendicular, there is usually no problem. Once you're in a safe site, depress the plunger steadily with moderate speed. If you push too hard or too fast, you can blow the syringe off the needle and lose the antibiotic. If you go too slowly, your horse might lose patience. It should take approximately 5 to 10 seconds to empty 20 cc into the horse's muscle.

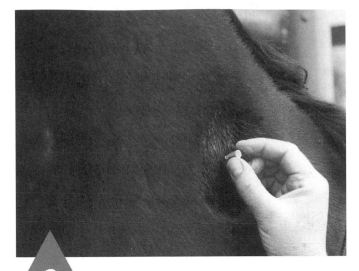

4 Withdraw the needle and syringe together in one careful but swift movement, pulling directly out in the same direction the needle went in — perpendicular to the horse's neck. Rub the spot to massage the liquid into the tissue and reestablish contact with your horse.

Safe and Healthy Techniques for Feeding

USING A HAY NET

A hay net is a plastic or cotton knotted rope web with a long drawstring that passes through metal rings at the top of the net. The drawstring is also used for tying the filled net to a wall, pen, or trailer. Although the holes in the net allow the horse to get at the hay, they also let hay fall on the ground, especially the flake from alfalfa hay.

To fill the hay net, lay the hay ration on the ground or on top of an intact bale of hay. Open the top of the hay net so the rings and drawstring make a large circle. Place the center of the bottom of the net on top of the hay ration. Let the rings and drawstring drape in a circle around the hay ration.

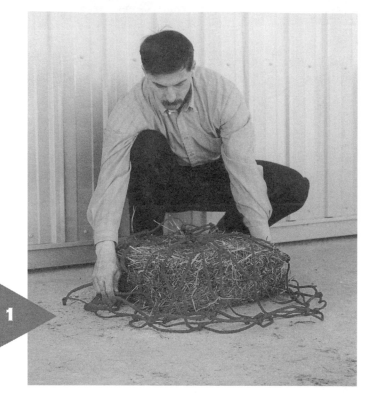

1

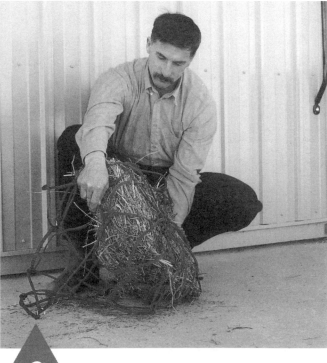

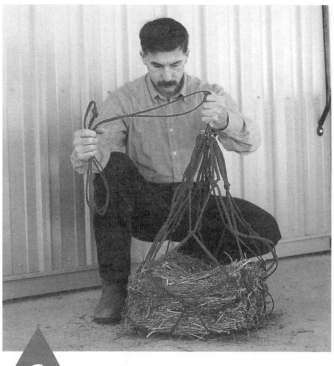

2 Place one hand on each side of the hay ration, lift up, and turn the pile and hay net over.

3 Now the hay net is upright with the hay inside. Pull on the drawstring to close the top of the net.

94

HANGING A HAY NET

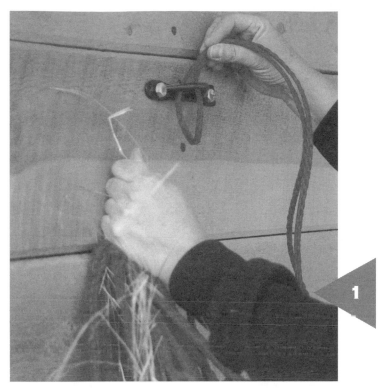

1 If you are going to use a hay net often, install a bracket or a heavy-duty screw eye on the stall wall at about 5'6" in height. Pass the hay net string through the bracket. Draw the hay net up until the top of the bag (where the rings are) is at the bracket.

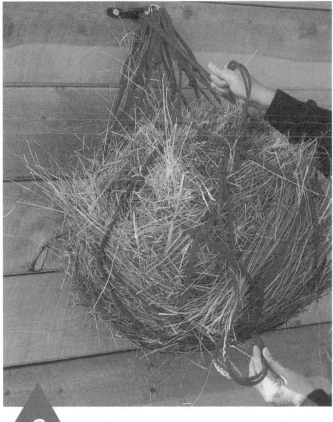

2 While you hold the bag in position with your right hand, use your left hand to weave the string back and forth through the squares of the net.

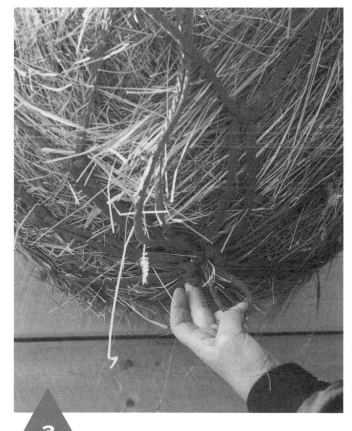

3 Then pass the end of the hay net string through the large ring at the bottom of the hay net.

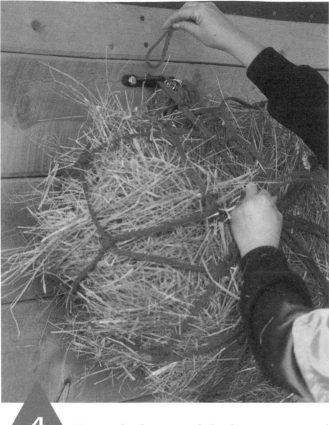

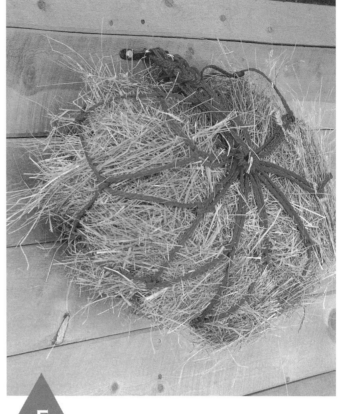

▲ 4   Draw the bottom of the hay net upward with your left hand while you feed the end of the string back through the bracket with your right hand.

▲ 5   Tie the hay string off with a quick-release knot with the end dropped through (see the Appendix for how to tie a quick-release knot). The net should be high and secure with no loose ends dangling.

HEIGHT TO HANG HAY NET

A hay net should be tied high enough so that when it is empty (and subsequently hangs lower) the horse cannot get a hoof or shoe caught in it.

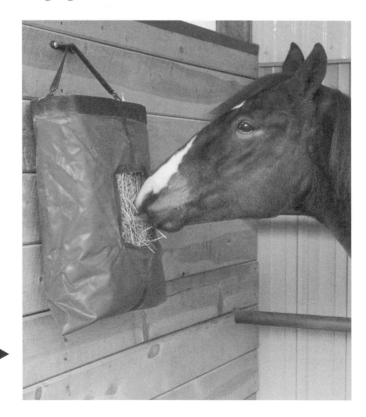

HAY BAG ▶

A hay bag is filled by simply sliding the hay into it and hanging it by its strap.

WEIGHING FEED

Each horse that you feed should have a specific ration that is designated by pounds of hay and pounds of various grains and supplements.

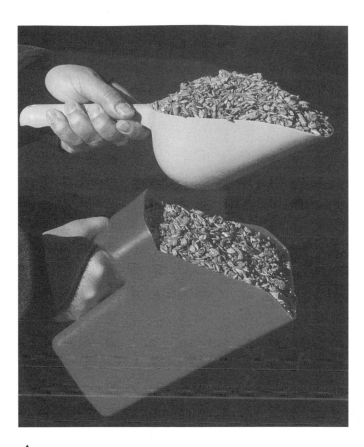

	AM	NOON	PM
Zipper	4# grass 4# alfalfa	2# wafers	Same as AM
Seeker	ditto	⊖	Same as AM
Drifter	2# grass 4# alfalfa	2# wafers 1 FF (oz) 1# Star Shine 1# g. vit-min 2# pellets	⊖	Same as AM
Zinger	4# grass 4# alfalfa	⊖	Same as AM
Aria	3# grass 4# alfalfa	2# wafers	Same as AM

▲

BLACKBOARD IN THE FEED ROOM

The best way to keep track of what each horse gets fed is to have a blackboard or an erasable board in the feed room. The board should list the ration for each feeding. In this case, some horses are fed three times a day.

▲

USE WEIGHT, NOT VOLUME

The reason it is so important to weigh feed is that the scoop method is very inaccurate. Both of these are scoops of respectable size, yet the one on the bottom holds twice the weight of grain as the top scoop. See how inaccurate it would be if you fed your horse "a scoop" of grain?

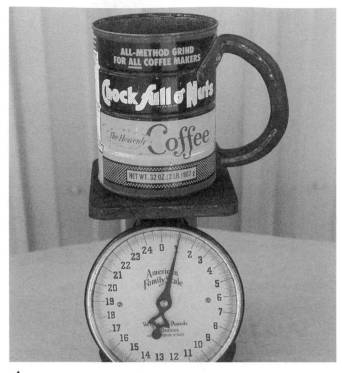

▲
MEASURE YOUR CONTAINER
Before you weigh the grain that you are going to feed your horse, you need to weigh your measuring container. This coffee can with custom horseshoe handle weighs about 1 pound.

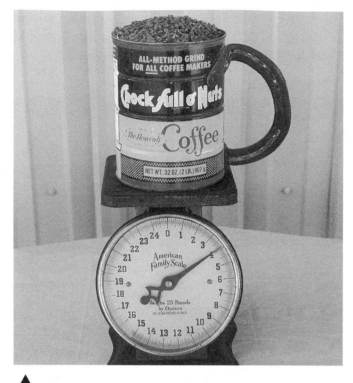

▲
WEIGHING PELLETED FEED
For example, when it is filled with a pelleted feed, the scale reads 3.9 pounds, so the can holds 2.9 pounds of pelleted feed. (When it is filled with a sweet feed, the scale reads 3.1 pounds, so the can holds 2.1 pounds of sweet feed.)

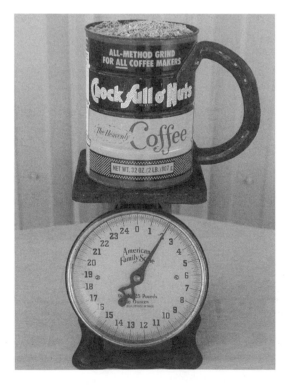

◄ WEIGHING BRAN
When it is filled with bran, the scale reads 2.1 pounds, so the can holds 1.1 pounds of bran.

WEIGHING HAY

The same thing goes for hay. All hay should be weighed. It should not just be fed by flakes. Which of the following hay rations looks like it weighs the most? Both examples are grass/alfalfa mix.

GRASS/ALFALFA MIX

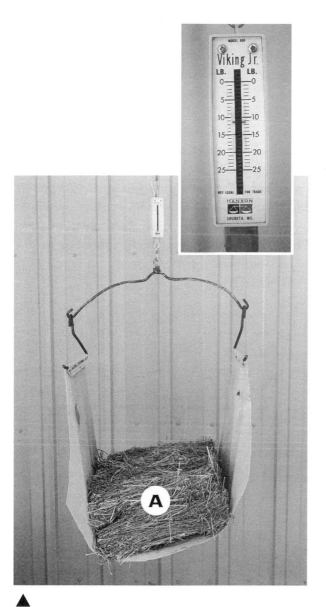

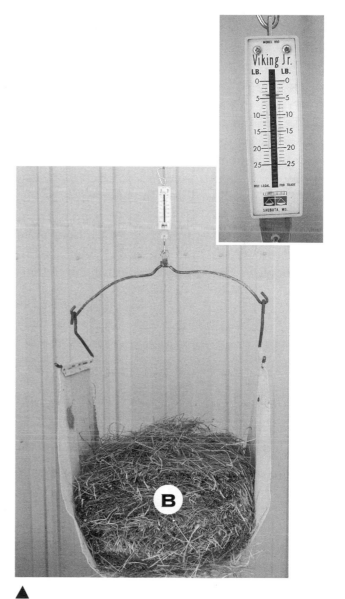

▲
DENSE FLAKES OF HAY
Let's look closer at the scales. Hay A, the smaller pile of hay, weighs 11.25 pounds. It is two flakes of dense, tightly packed, leafy hay.

▲
LOOSE FLAKES OF HAY
Hay B, the larger pile of hay, weighs 4.1 pounds. It is two flakes of loose, fluffy hay made up of fine, immature stems.

Making a Mash

If a horse is old or ill or has dental problems, there might be merit in feeding him a mash. A mash is basically a horse porridge. It is a mixture of grain and hot water and other ingredients. The mix is steamed, then allowed to cool somewhat before feeding to the horse. A mash is easy for a horse to chew and digest because the fibrous grain hulls and particles are softened.

For years, the most popular mash for horses has been bran mash, but feeding large amounts of bran regularly to a horse can actually harm the horse. Bran contains large amounts of the mineral phosphorus, which binds with the calcium in a horse's diet, preventing him from absorbing the calcium. When a horse does not absorb enough calcium, the bones might become weakened, and in some instances, the weakened bones bulge. Therefore, young horses should rarely if ever be fed bran. In addition, there may be an increase in the likelihood of a horse developing enteroliths (intestinal "stones") if you make it a point to feed him bran on a regular basis.

You can make a mash out of almost any grain product that your horse is accustomed to eating: oats, barley, corn, and sweet feed mixtures. Whereas whole grains won't absorb as much water as finely flaked feed such as bran, whole grains will swell and soften and provide a warm, soft feed for horses that require it. Pelleted feed will readily soften and turn to mush, so if you plan to utilize them in the mash, take care not to add too much water or your horse will refuse the resulting "soup."

You can also experiment and add special ingredients to entice your ill or old horse to eat and drink: salt, molasses, carrot slices, apple slices, and so on. When you add things to the mash, start with small amounts at first (e.g., 1 teaspoon of salt or ½ cup of carrots), and increase as your horse gets used to them. Contrary to what you might think, there are some horses that just don't like carrots or refuse feed with molasses in it.

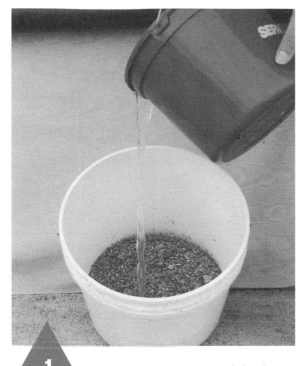

1 Put the horse's normal feed ration in a bucket. Add HOT water (boiling water is best but very hot tap water will also work) to the grain mixture so that the feed is wet but not covered with water. You will have to experiment somewhat with the ratio of water to grain, depending on the texture of the grain ration. Start with a ratio of 2 parts grain to 1 part water.

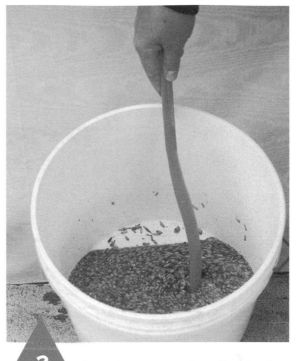

2 Stir the mixture briefly. A clean sweat scraper works well for this.

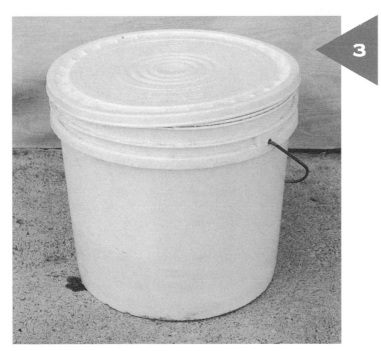

3 Cover the pail and let it steam for 5 or 10 minutes. Be sure the mash has cooled to a safe temperature. The best way to check is to plunge your hand into the pail. If it is a comfortable temperature, you can use your mash-covered hand to scoop the bran out of the steaming bucket and into the horse's regular grain feeder. Be sure to wash the steaming bucket so it's ready to use. If you feed your horse a mash, you will also have to wash his regular grain feeder daily. Remove all mash from your horse's feeder that he has not consumed within 2 hours after feeding. (Wet feed spoils much faster than dry feed.)

FEEDING MANNERS

Even though horses are very hungry at feeding time, they should show good manners when you feed them. They should not rush at you or crowd you. If each *horse is taught good manners singly, they will be much more likely to be safely fed as a group.*

IN THE BARN

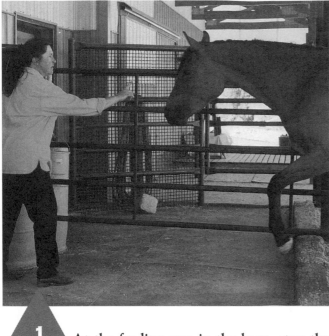

1 At the feeding area in the barn, stop the horse at the edge with a verbal command, "WHOA," used with body language. After he has stopped, tell him to "WAIT" and give him a signal with an outstretched hand as well.

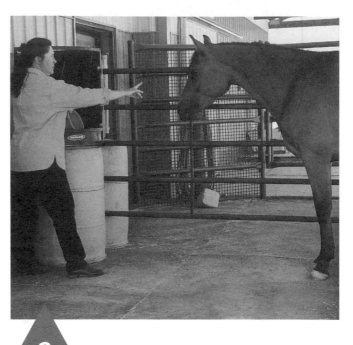

2 Place the grain in the feeder but continue to tell the horse to "WAIT" at the edge of the feeding area.

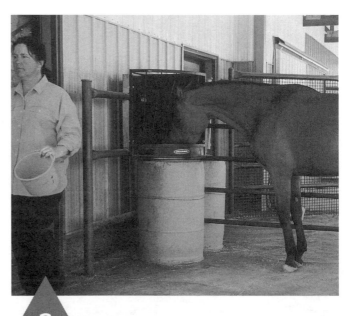

3 Tell him he can come to the feeder by using the verbal command "OK!"

In the Pasture

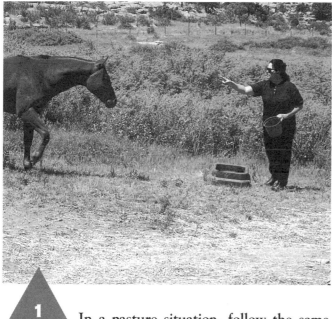

1 In a pasture situation, follow the same procedure. First, stop the horse with the voice command "WHOA."

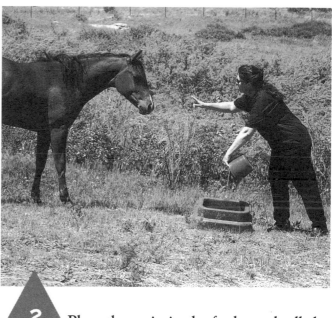

2 Place the grain in the feeder and tell the horse to "WAIT" — with words and a hand signal.

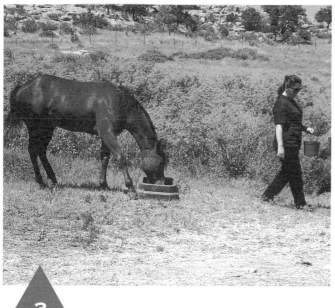

3 Tell the horse "OK," and allow the horse to move in to eat.

Protective Equipment for Your Horse

Your horse's legs and feet are very important to his comfort and function. There are various instances when the limbs need the extra protection of equipment such as protective boots, bandages, exercise wraps, stable wraps, and shipping wraps. Protective equipment should always be chosen carefully, well fitted, and properly adjusted.

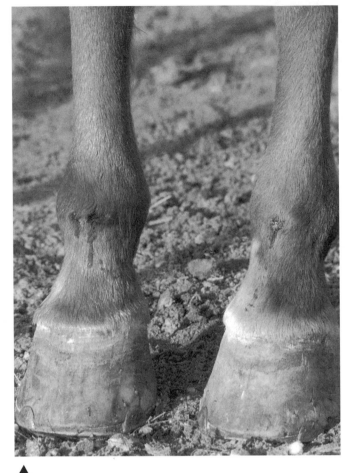

▲
OPEN SORES
This horse has developed open sores on the fronts of her fetlocks from the act of lying down and getting up on hard, dry pasture.

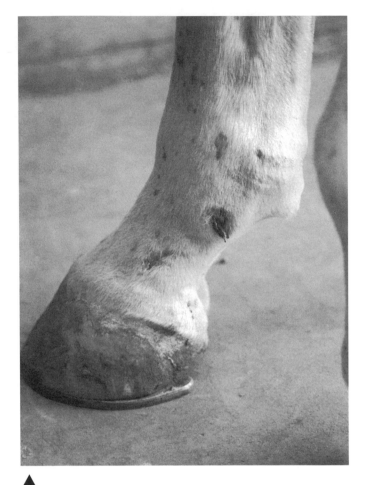

▲
INTERFERENCE
This horse hits himself as he works. These are interference marks.

PROTECTIVE BOOTS

Most manufacturers offer boots in at least two or three sizes. "Standard" or "Medium" fits most 1000- to 1100-pound saddle horses. Most boots are designed to be worn snugly. Boots that are adjusted too loosely move around on the horse's leg, allow dirt to enter, can cause abrasions, hinder movement, or injure tendons. Boots that are made of neoprene (closed cell foam) are designed for short-term application (2 hours or less), as they concentrate heat and cause sweating.

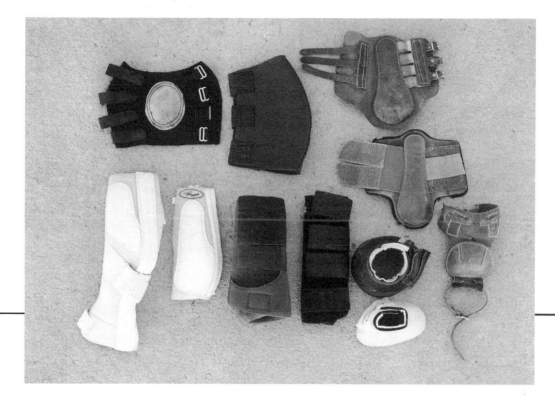

TYPES OF PROTECTIVE BOOTS

There are various types of protective boots available. *Clockwise from upper left:* Fetlock boots prevent sores on the fronts of the fetlocks; hock boots prevent sores on the outsides of the hocks. All-leather splint boots protect the inside of the lower limb from being injured by the opposite limb; synthetic splint boots with a hard plastic plate protect the inside of the lower limb. Rundown or skid boots protect the ergot/rear fetlock area when a reining, cutting, or roping horse stops deep and hard. Two types of bell boots, which encircle the coronary band, protect it from blows when the horse is working or traveling in a trailer. Three types of sport boots offer elastic support to flexor tendons and protection to the inside of the limb. There is also a combination sport boot/bell boot available.

SPORT BOOT

The purpose of support boots is to support the limb and its structures.

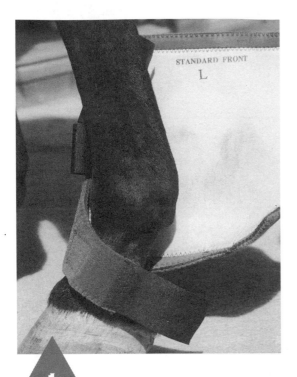

1 Fit the sport boot to the contours of the horse's limb.

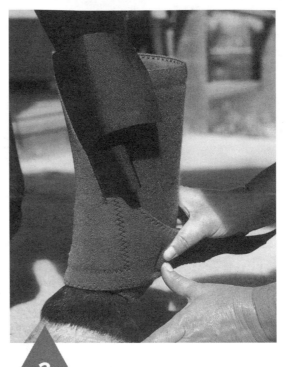

2 Lightly tack the bottom strap in place to keep it out of the way. If you start by fastening the bottom first, the top almost never comes out even.

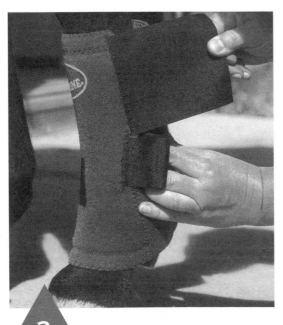

3 Attach the top strap first, so you can line up the top edges.

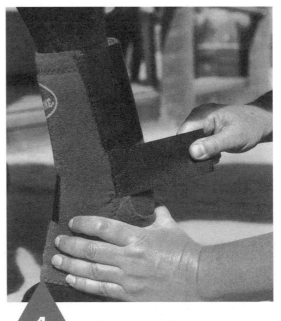

4 Pull the stretchy straps tight, so that the boots conform to the horse's limb. You might have to refasten the straps several times before the boot is tight enough. If too loose, the boots could cause raw spots.

SPLINT BOOT

Splint books have a thick and/or hard plate for the inside of the leg so the leg is protected from blows *by the other hoof. This type of classic splint boot has elastic strips attached to the buckles.*

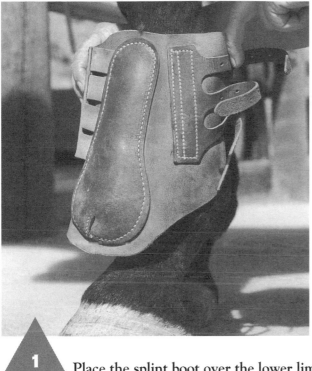

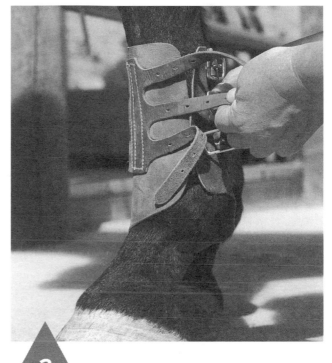

1 Place the splint boot over the lower limb.

2 Locate the protective plate on the inside of the limb and buckle the straps on the outside.

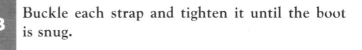

3 Buckle each strap and tighten it until the boot is snug.

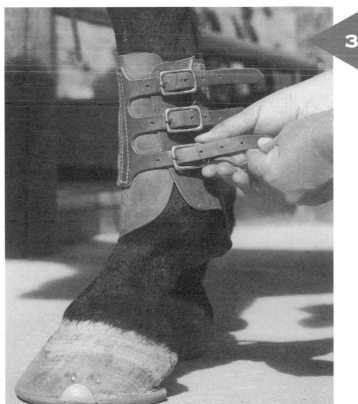

BELL BOOT

The bell boot encircles the coronary band to protect it from blows when the horse is working or traveling in a trailer.

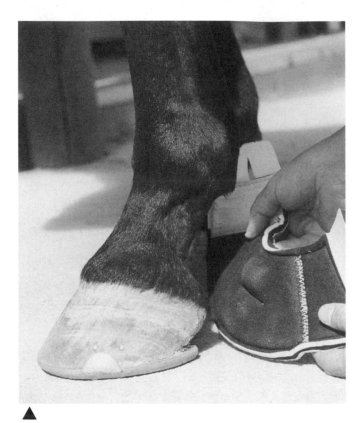

▲
FITTING THE PASTERN
This bell boot is designed to fit the contours of the horse's pastern and heel area. The protrusion in the neoprene is designed to fit into the depression at the base of the pastern to lock the boot in place.

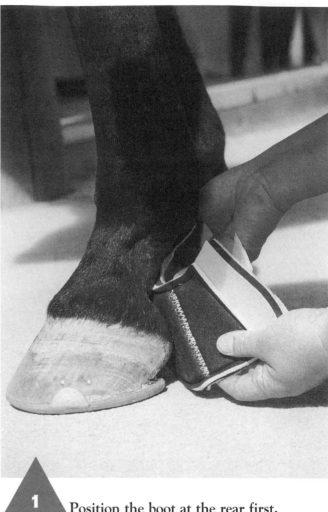

1 Position the boot at the rear first.

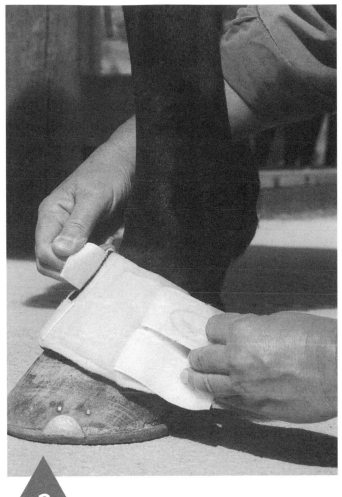

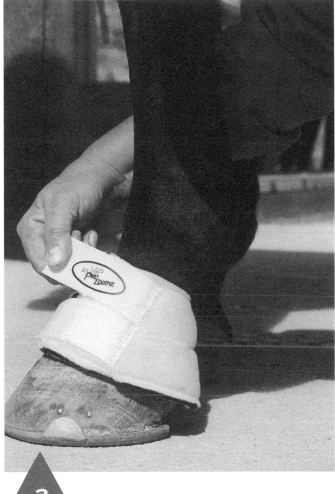

2 Bring the two sides of the boots together at the front of the hoof. Fasten the first set of hook-and-loop closures while you hold the top set out of the way.

3 Fasten the top layer of hook-and-loop closures in a double-lock fastening. This is essential for the boots to stay on when the horse is working.

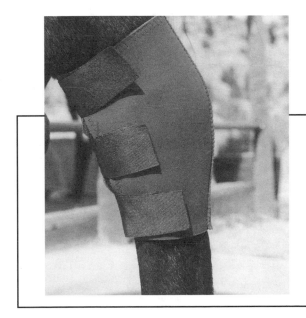

PROTECTIVE HOCK BOOT

This shows a protective hock boot in proper position. Some horses get chronic sores on the outside of their hocks when they lie down or roll. These boots protect the hocks from abrasions. However, because these boots are made of neoprene, they can be used only for short periods of time.

BANDAGES

ROLLING A BANDAGE

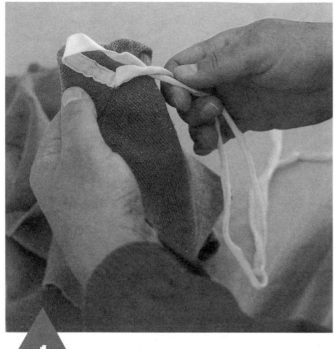

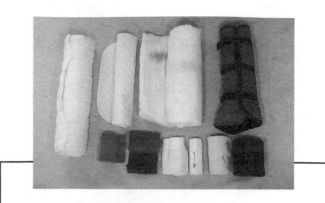

TYPES OF BANDAGES: *(from left top row)* 17" x 30" washable polyester padding with hook-and-loop closure, 12" x 30" washable cotton leg quilt, 14" x 30" disposable cotton batting, fleece-lined nylon travel boot; (bottom row from left) 4" x 15' elastic crepe bandage, 4" x 9' cotton track wrap with cotton ties, 4" stretchy crepe, 5" cotton bandage with pin, 5" flannel bandage with pin, 4¾" x 9' polar fleece track wrap with hook-and-loop closures.

1 To roll a bandage, with the bandage laundered and dried, pick up the end with the tie strings.

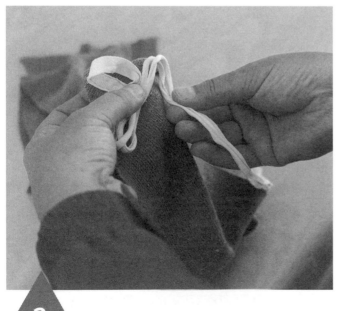

2 Hold the bandage with the side where the strings are attached facing you. Fold the strings back and forth.

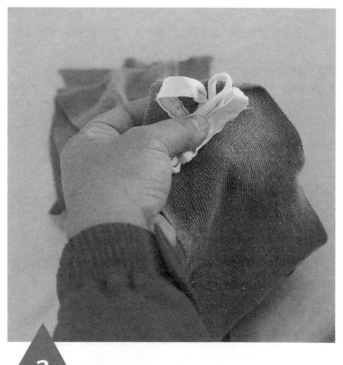

3 Once you have them all in a neat pile, you are ready to begin rolling.

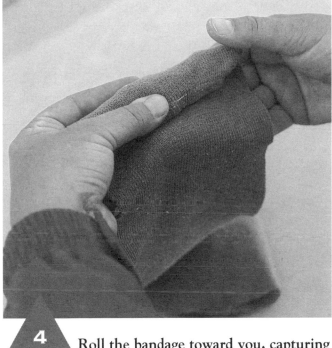

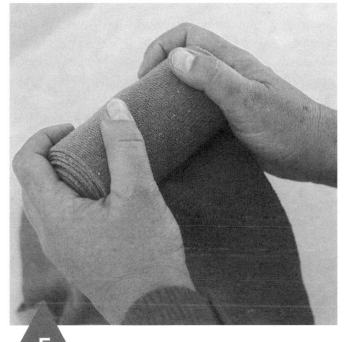

4 Roll the bandage toward you, capturing the strings inside the bandage. If you have bandages with hook-and-loop closures, fold the hook strip onto the same side of the bandages as the loop strip and roll the bandage up with both strips on the inside.

5 Continue rolling, keeping the sides of the bandage roll even by holding it between your hands like this.

◀ BANDAGE ROLLER
An alternative to hand-rolling is using a bandage-roller.

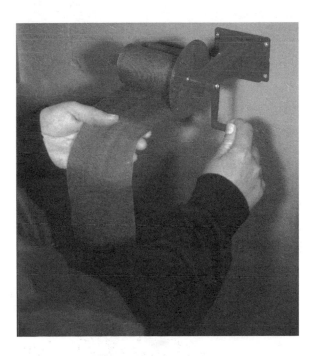

Applying an Exercise Wrap

An exercise wrap is designed to support and protect the tendons of a horse's lower limb when he is working during training or when he is playing hard during turnout. The uses and functions of well-applied exercise wraps and support boots are similar. The type of bandage used for an exercise wrap can range from non-stretchy knit cotton that has minimal give, to fluffy, stretchy polar fleece, to sport bandages with a moderate amount of elastic. Since exercise wraps are put on quite tight, even though for short periods of time, it is essential that the tension is appropriate, even, and smooth. It is a good idea to use a very thin leg pad underneath an exercise wrap to help equalize the distribution of pressure. (See **Which Way to Wrap?**, p. 117, for more on applying an exercise wrap.)

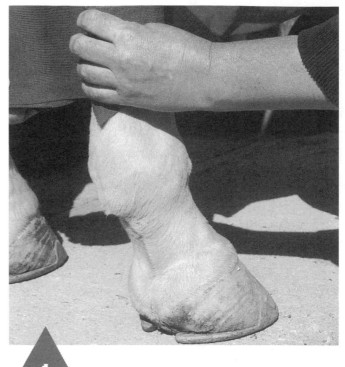

1 Be sure when you start unrolling the bandage that you will have the tape ties or hook-and-loop closure on the outside when you are finished (see **Bandages**, p. 110), otherwise you will have no way to fasten the wrap. Take care not to begin the bandage on the rear (flexor tendons) or the front (extensor tendons) of the limb because the bandage end could cause the tendons to become sore. Instead, position the bandage end in the middle of the inside or outside of the leg. Start in the middle of the cannon. Keep the tension firm and even.

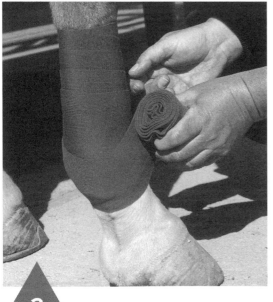

2 Wrap down until you get to the fetlock and then cradle it in a sling.

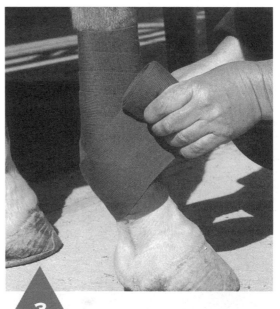

3 Wrap around the fetlock once more. Bring the bandage upward, so the support forms an **X** at the rear of the fetlock. Wrap upward.

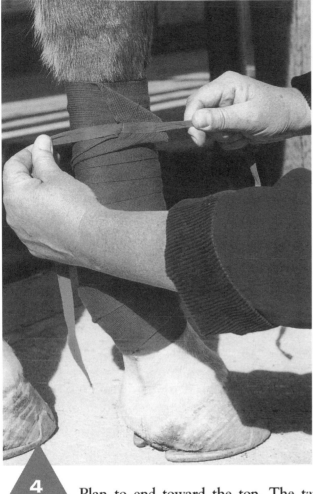

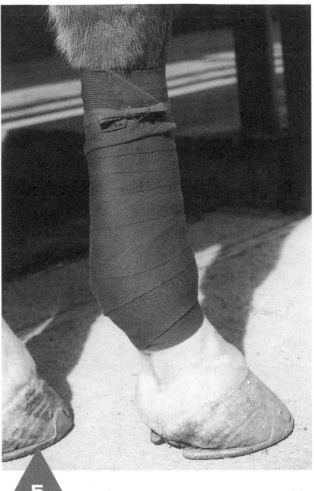

4 Plan to end toward the top. The tapes should be on the outside of the bandage.

5 Tie the cotton tapes in a knot and bow. Secure the bow by tucking the ends underneath the ties. Some people like to place a piece of adhesive tape over the bow.

◀ THE **X** SUPPORT

This front view shows the **X** support at the rear forming a corresponding **X** support in the front.

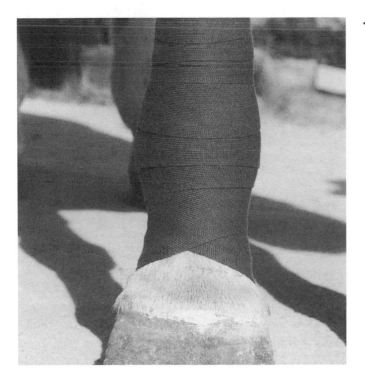

Applying a Stable Wrap

A stable wrap, also called a standing bandage, is somewhat like a wound bandage without the salve, dressing, and gauze. It is a piece of quilting that is held in place with a roll bandage. A stable wrap is sometimes used with liniment to reduce swelling and fluid accumulation in the lower limb. The horse's legs are rubbed and wrapped before he is put in the stall at night. A stable wrap should be removed for at least an hour every 12–16 hours.

Leg Quilts

Choose appropriate padding. Leg quilts come in various materials with coverings commonly of cotton, polyester, or flannel and fillings of cotton batting, polyester fiberfill, and foam. Quilts of cotton batting and a cotton/polyester cover are my favorite. Foam quilts are too warm. Sizes range from 12" to 18" tall and from 30" to 42" wide. Average for front legs is 12" or 14" x 30"; for hinds 14" or 16" x 30".

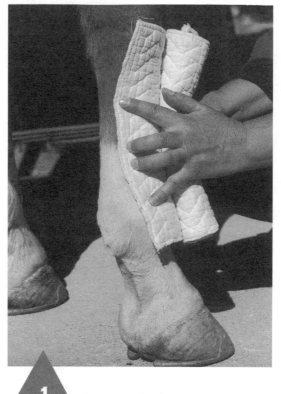

1 Start with the edge of the quilt on one side of the leg or the other, not on the front or back of the limb.

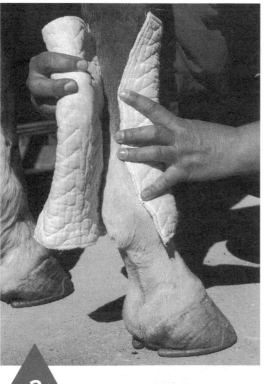

2 Unroll the quilt, holding the beginning edge in position. Don't put the starting edge of the quilt over the flexor tendon area or the thick edge might cause the horse discomfort by morning.

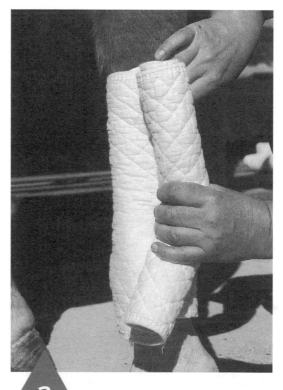

3 This is about the perfect height for a quilt on this horse's leg. Note: Wrapping a quilt too tall will cause interference with the knee, which would make it impossible to get a good, smooth fit.

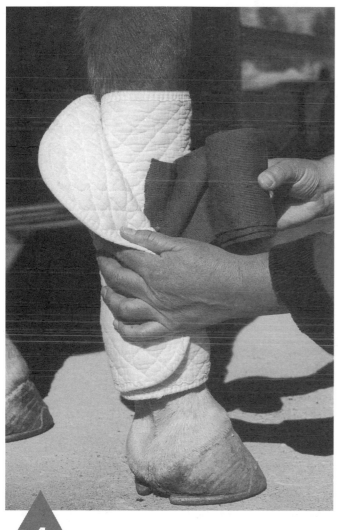

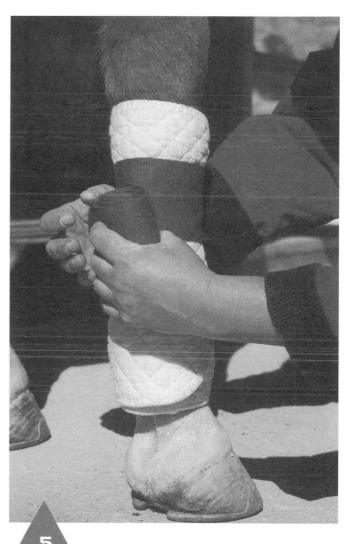

4 Choose a wider and longer bandage than the exercise wrap. Bandages for stable and shipping wraps are customarily 5" to 6" wide and up to 12' long. One way to start the bandage is to place the end of the bandage underneath the edge of the quilt. Simply unroll your bandage in the same direction you unrolled the quilt. If you did the opposite, you'd be loosening and "unscrewing" the quilt.

5 If you know your bandages and your horse's leg, you can start out this high, but if your bandage is not wide enough or long enough or if your horse's cannon is very long, you might not have enough bandage to go all the way down, back up again, and finish.

As you are working your way back up, keep the tension even and the wraps as symmetrical as possible. When you get to the top, decide where you will place the ties.

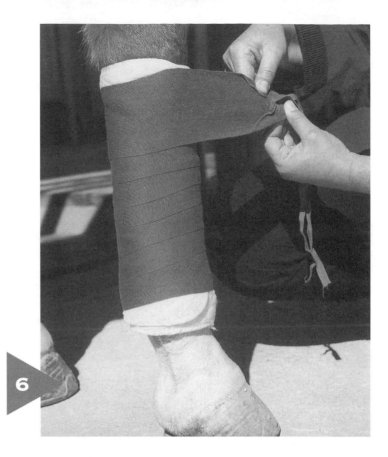

6

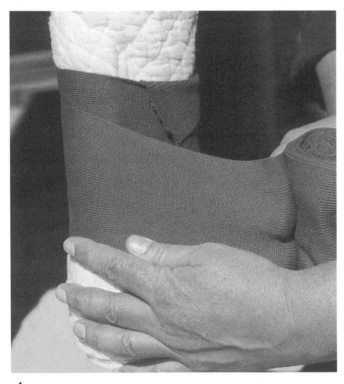

▲
ALTERNATIVE METHOD FOR STARTING BANDAGE

Another way to start a bandage is to fold an ear over to lock the bandage in place.

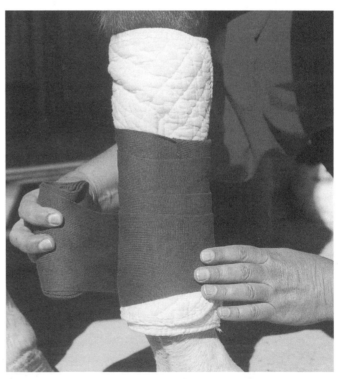

▲
ALTERNATIVE FOR STARTING MID-CANNON

This is a more customary starting point: mid-cannon. Note: If this leg quilt had ended on the inside of the leg, the final edge of the leg quilt would face backward, which would be more desirable.

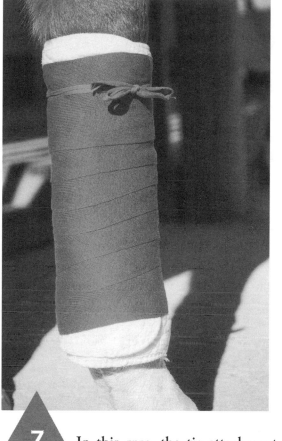

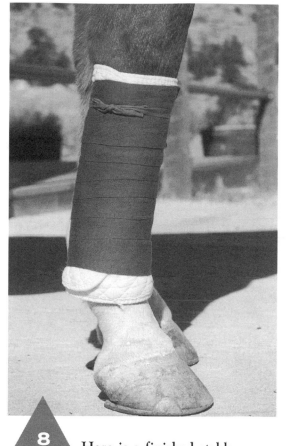

7 In this case, the tie attachments are on the inside of the leg and the ties have been wrapped around to the outside of the leg.

8 Here is a finished stable wrap, with the bow tucked underneath the strings.

WHICH WAY TO WRAP

You may have heard that there is only one correct direction to wrap a horse's leg. In fact, it does not matter whether you bandage clockwise or counterclockwise; either way, you have to bring the bandage alternately from front to back and then from back to front. Depending on which leg you are bandaging, and whether you are right- or left-handed, one direction might be easier for you to wrap properly than the other.

What does matter is that you develop a feel for an even tension throughout the bandage. Have an experienced horseman check your bandaging technique until you are confident that you have mastered the skills.

1. Never exert strong pressure on the flexor tendons (at the back of the leg) or pull them to the side, because that could lead to tendon problems.
2. Don't pull strongly across the extensor tendons at the front of the horse's cannon.
3. Always wrap the bandage in the same direction as the quilt.
4. Be sure there are no lumps or wrinkles in the quilt or bandage.
5. Use an even tension that is appropriate for the specific bandage and the type of bandaging material you are using.

APPLYING A SHIPPING WRAP

A *shipping wrap*, also called a travel or trailer wrap, is designed to protect a horse during trailering. For a travel wrap, you will need tall quilts that extend from the knee to the coronary band and a wide, long bandage.

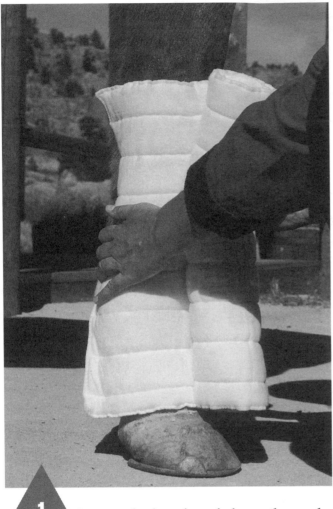

1 Start with the edge of the quilt on the inside of the cannon.

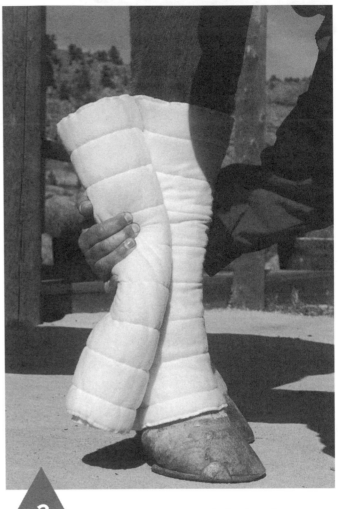

2 Wrap the quilt around the leg, keeping it snug and low on the leg.

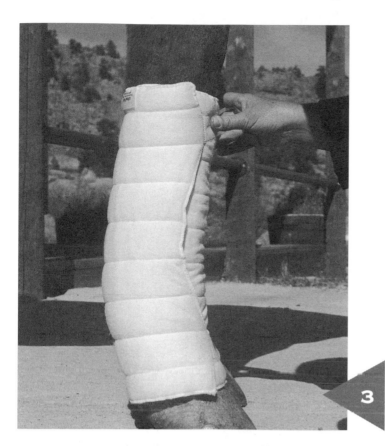

▶ 3 Fasten the hook-and-loop closures that will hold the quilt in place while you begin wrapping.

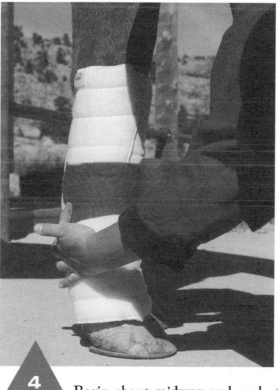

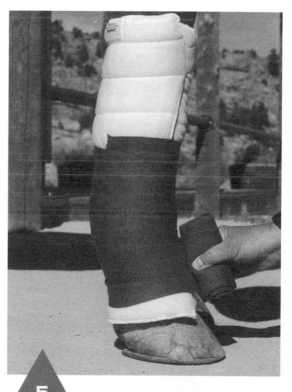

▲ 4   Begin about midway and apply the bandage in the same direction as you did the quilt. Because you are wrapping over a thicker quilt and a longer area, if you are using a 4" x 9' bandage like this one, you will have to use it very efficiently or there will not be enough to finish. A 6" x 12' bandage would be better.

▲ 5   Wrap down to the coronary band, leaving some quilt extending out the bottom.

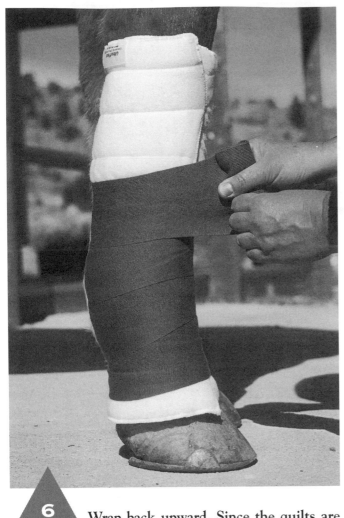

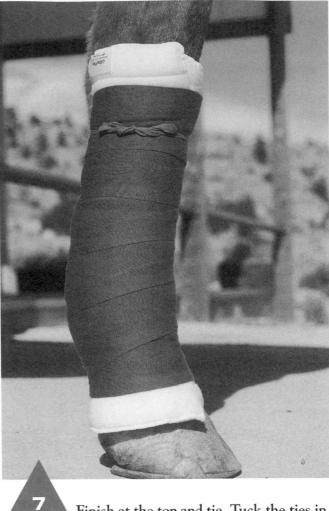

6 Wrap back upward. Since the quilts are very thick, you can apply quite a bit of tension as you wrap. If you don't, you will probably find the bandage on the trailer floor.

7 Finish at the top and tie. Tuck the ties in.

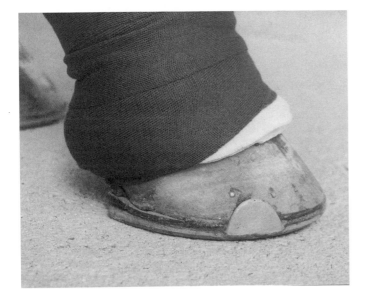

◀ **INCREASED PROTECTION**

To positively protect the bulbs of the heels, you can place a bell boot over the bottom portion of the bandage. But you will need a larger size bell boot for this purpose than the ones you use on your horse for exercise. A bell boot will not only protect the bulbs of the heels and further protect the coronary band, but it will also keep the lower portion of the bandage from getting dirty or ripped. An alternative to the bell boot is to end both the quilt and wrap much farther down on the hoof, such as shown here.

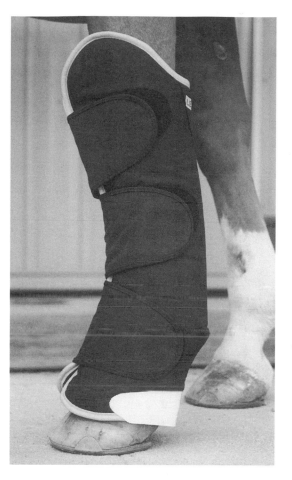

◀ TRAVELING BOOTS

Instead of applying traveling wraps, you can use one of many types of traveling boots, such as these heavy nylon boots. To offer extra protection if a horse were to step up onto the bulbs of the heels with a hind hoof, the bottom of these boots is reinforced with a heavy plastic scuff plate.

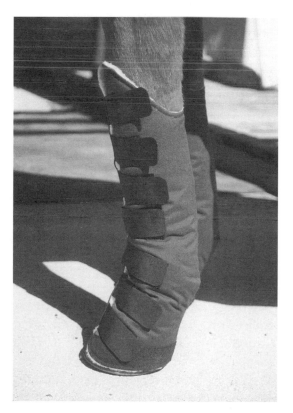

◀ SHIPPING BOOTS

These tall shipping boots are well padded and have Kevlar sewn to the bottom. Kevlar is the material used in bulletproof vests, so it will withstand the abuse from the other hooves.

Horse Clothing

MEASURING A HORSE FOR A BLANKET

Choosing the correct sheet or blanket size depends on the measurement directions suggested by the manufacturer. The most common instructions for blanket or sheet measurement are as follows.

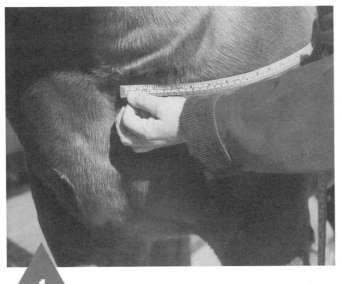

1 Begin by standing the horse squarely. Hold the end of the measuring tape at the center of the horse's chest, and measure around the widest part of the shoulder.

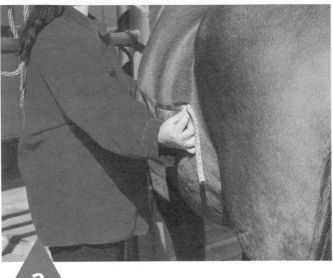

2 Continue along the barrel . . .

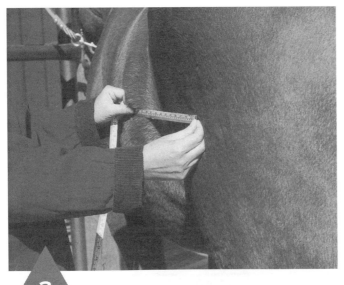

3 . . . keeping your tape horizontal. (Most 60" tape measures end at the flank, so you will need to note your spot and begin the tape again.)

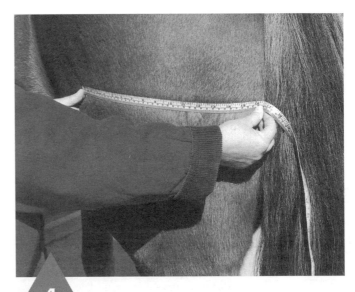

4 Go around the widest part of the hindquarter to the edge of the tail (or mid-thigh). Keep the measuring tape horizontal. The number of inches indicates what size sheet the horse should wear. If the measurement is an odd number, use the next highest even measurement.

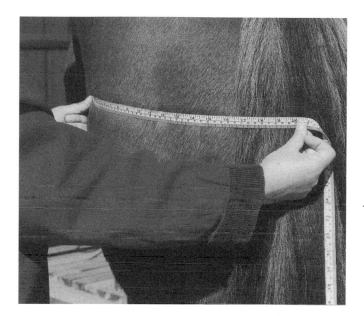

◀ VARIATION: MEASURE TO
CENTER OF TAIL

Some manufacturers say to measure to the center of
the tail. But the difference between mid-thigh and tail
center can be as much as 6 inches, which could make
a blanket fit great or poorly.

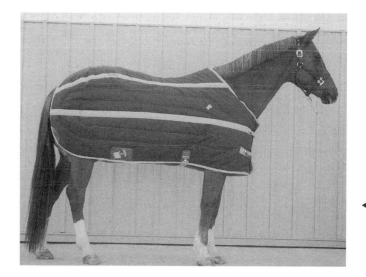

◀ A GOOD FIT

This 1200-pound, 16-hand gelding measures 79"
to the edge of his tail and this size-80 blanket fits
him well.

TYPES OF HORSE CLOTHING

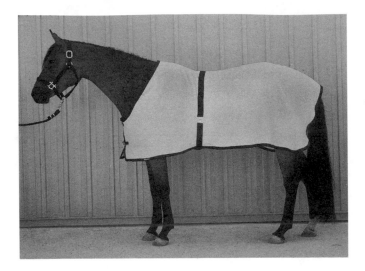

◀ ANTI-SWEAT SHEET
Made of open-mesh fibers, such as cotton, which tend to wick sweat and cool a horse and also prevent him from sweating. Some anti-sweat sheets double as fly sheets. Solid, synthetic anti-sweat sheets are a new innovation.

Use in very hot weather. Not suitable for a turn-out sheet because it usually has no leg straps and can easily slip or be torn.

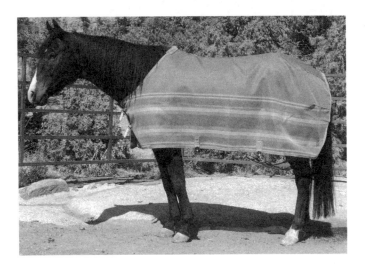

◀ FLY SHEET
Made of open-mesh materials, such as nylon or polyester, that keep flies from landing and biting. Some models are durable enough for turnout.

Use instead of fly spray during times of particularly heavy fly infestations.

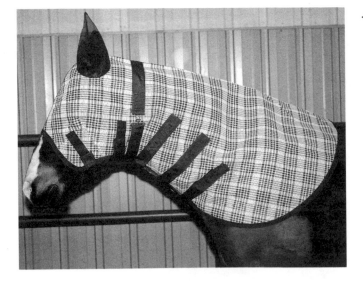

◀ FLY HOOD
Made of open-mesh material with protection from flies for the eyes and ears as well.

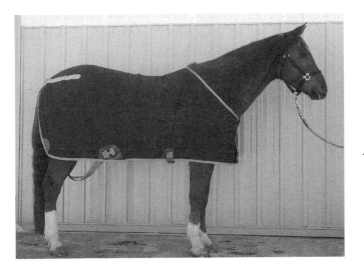

◀ STABLE SHEET

Made of light material, such as cotton. Unlined except for shoulder area. Mainly to keep dust and dirt off horse's coat. May or may not have leg straps, but *not* designed for turnout.

Used in stall to keep horse clean.

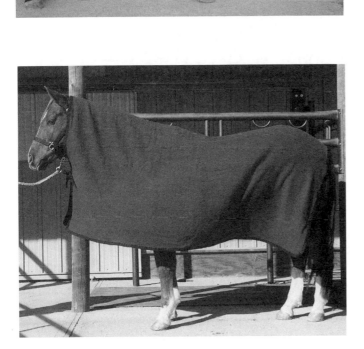

◀ TURN-OUT SHEET

Made of more durable fabrics, such as Cordura, or nylon, or cotton canvas. Unlined except for shoulder area. May or may not be water repellent or water resistant. Usually has leg straps to prevent sheet from twisting when horse rolls or runs.

Used in pens, paddocks, or pastures on horses that are turned out for exercise. May or may not be machine washable; some will need to be hosed and brushed.

◀ COOLER

Made of wool, wool blends, or polyester fleece. Unfitted style to drape over horse from poll to tail to wick moisture off wet horse and allow him to cool out gradually without becoming chilled.

Used on horses after bathing or hard work. Horse must be tied in cross-ties or stall, or the cooler will certainly be damaged.

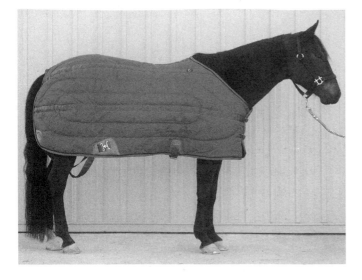

◀ STABLE BLANKET

Made of warm yet lightweight materials. Either the blanket is lined with blanket-type material or entire blanket is quilted with polyester batting and lined with nylon. Not designed to be waterproof.

Used on stalled horses to keep them warm. Usually suitable for temperatures below 45°F or the horse will sweat. Machine washable in a triple-load washing machine.

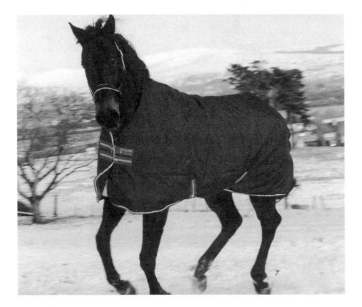

◀ TURN-OUT BLANKET

Made of warm, very tough, weather-resistant materials. Often the outer shell is waterproof or water resistant. The filling and lining can be of the similar materials as the stable blanket. Has leg straps.

Used on horses in pens, paddocks, and pastures during cold weather. Might be machine washable but might require hosing and brushing.

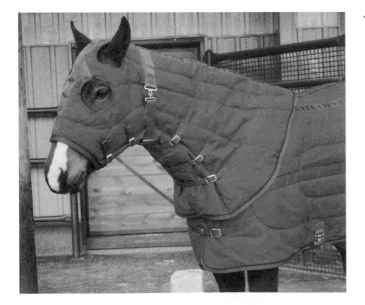

◀ HOOD

Usually designed to go along with stable blanket or turn-out blanket to provide total protection for the neck and head during cold weather.

Used on (show) horses that have been body clipped or are kept blanketed year-round.

PUTTING ON AN OPEN-FRONT BLANKET

An open-front blanket is one that has buckles in the front, which allows the blanket to be adjusted.

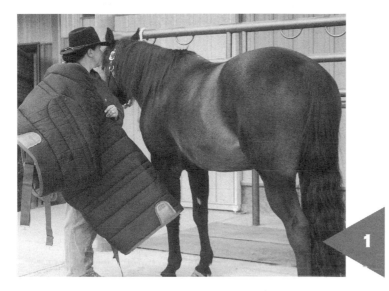

1 To put it on a horse, turn the blanket inside out. It should be folded in half, back to front.

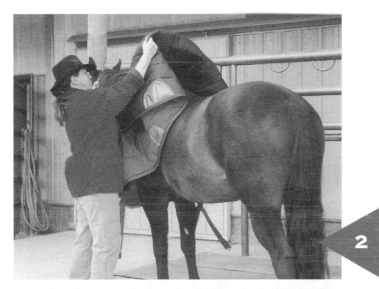

2 Place the blanket on the front of the horse, slightly ahead of where it will lie.

2A ALTERNATIVELY: If your horse is accustomed to blanketing, you can throw the blanket into place.

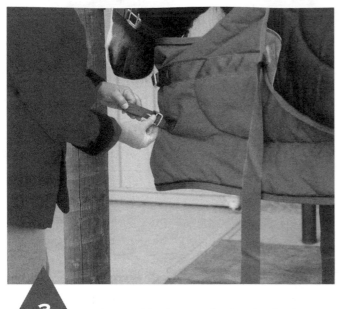

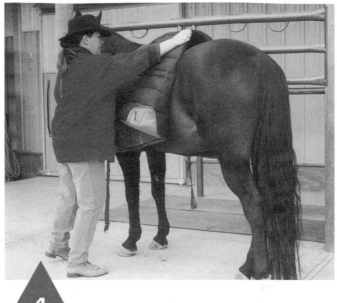

▲ **3** With the blanket well ahead of where it will eventually rest, buckle the front straps at the chest.

▲ **4** Then pull the blanket back into position with it still folded in half.

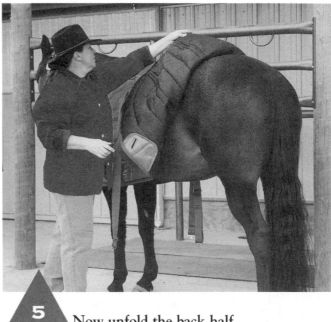

▲ **5** Now unfold the back half.

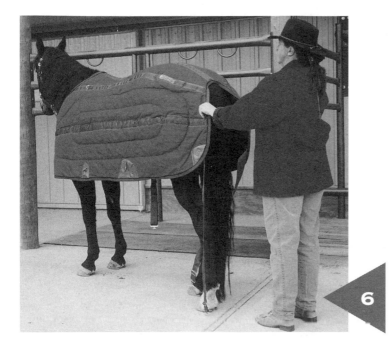

6 Stand behind your horse and straighten the blanket so that the midline of the blanket goes directly down the center of his back.

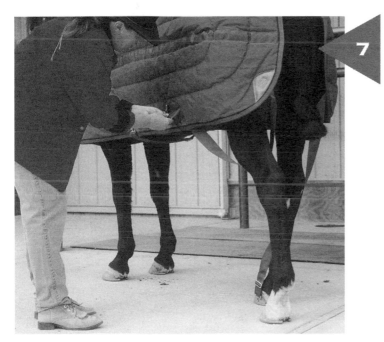

7 Buckle the front *surcingle*, which is the strap that encircles the heart girth. The adjustment and attachment of the hind leg straps is important. If hind leg straps are adjusted too short, every time the horse moves or turns, the action of the hind legs pulls the blanket backward, putting pressure on the horse's shoulder. Leg straps that are adjusted too short often rip off the blanket. If the straps are adjusted too long, the horse can get tangled in them when stomping at flies, lying down, or rolling. To prevent the straps from rubbing the hair off the thin skin on the inside of a horse's legs, there are two methods of attachment.

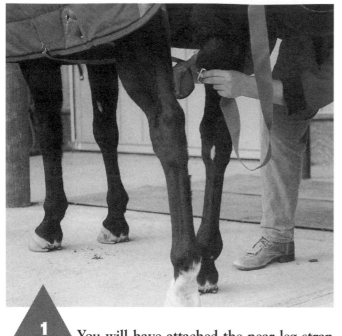

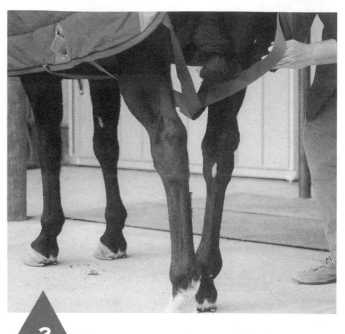

1 You will have attached the near leg strap to the blanket on the near side. Go to the off side. Take the off strap and run it through the near strap once. Then attach it to the off side.

2 This creates an **X** between the horse's legs and holds the straps away from the insides of the horse's legs.

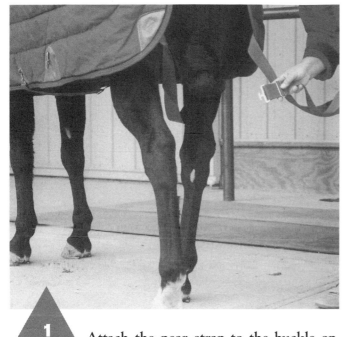

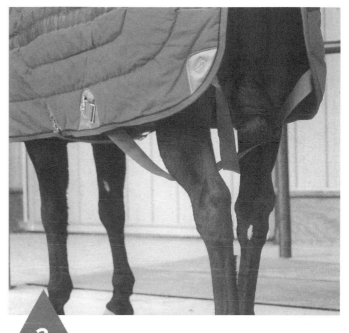

1 Attach the near strap to the buckle on the off side of the blanket. You have created a diagonal line with the strap.

2 Now take the off side strap and attach it to the buckle on the near side. You have created an X between the horse's legs. The style and position of the fasteners, and the blanket design and fit, will dictate which of these methods will work best for you.

PUTTING ON A CLOSED-FRONT BLANKET OR SHEET

A closed-front blanket has a solid front that cannot be unbuckled. This means the blanket has to be put on over the horse's head.

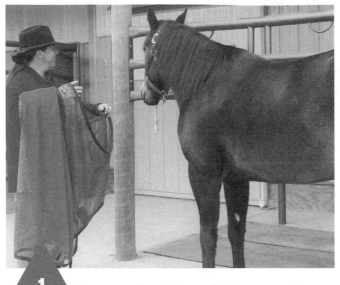

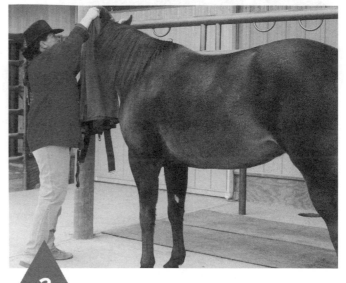

1 To put a closed-front fly sheet on a horse, tie him to a tie rail. Put your right arm through the sheet from back to front. Your right hand will come out at the wither area of the sheet. Unsnap the lead rope from the halter.

2 Hold the halter with your left hand as you slide the sheet off your right arm onto the horse's head. Remember that the wither area of the sheet will go on the horse's head last.

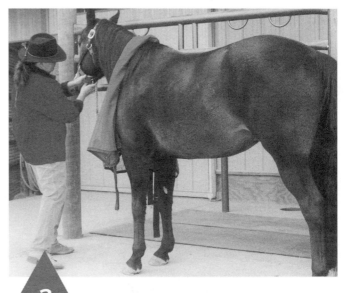

3 Leave the sheet hanging around your horse's neck. Snap the lead rope back to the halter.

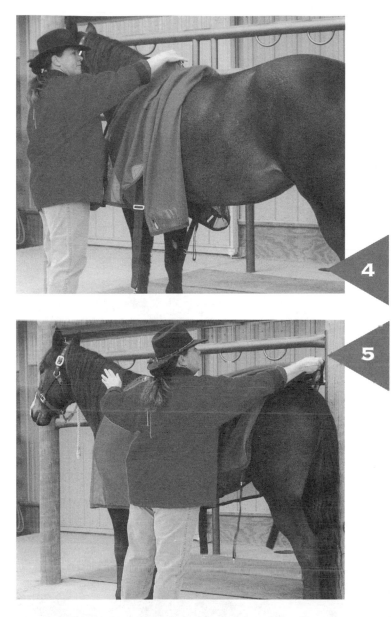

4 Position the sheet and begin unfolding it.

5 Keeping the sheet centered on your horse's back, draw it back to the hindquarters.

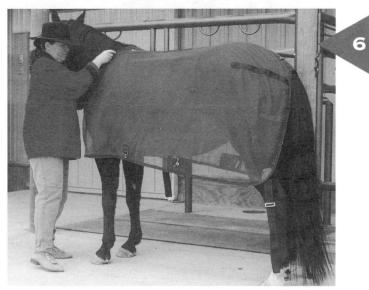

6 Position the front. Buckle the front surcingle and hind leg straps as indicated with the open-front blanket (see pp. 129–131).

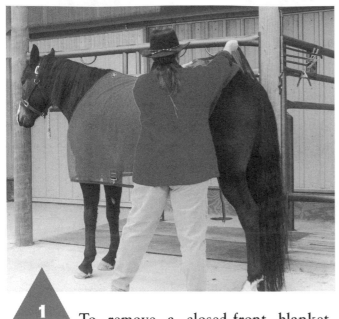

1 To remove a closed-front blanket, reverse the process. Start by unbuckling the hind leg straps and front surcingle. Lift up the sheet from the hindquarters.

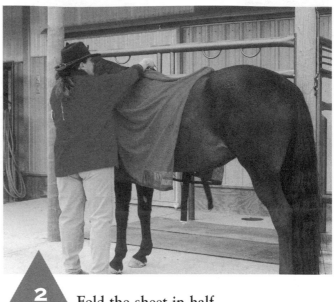

2 Fold the sheet in half.

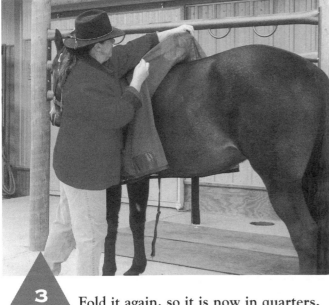

3 Fold it again, so it is now in quarters.

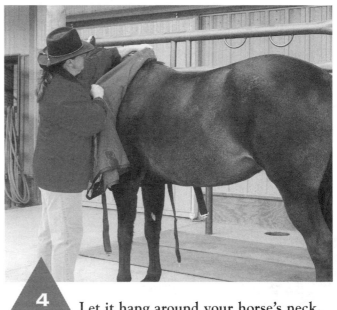

4 Let it hang around your horse's neck.

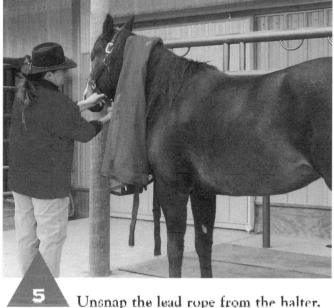

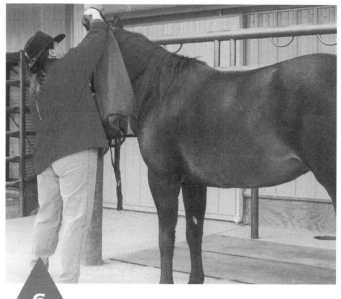

5 ▲ Unsnap the lead rope from the halter.

6 ▲ Lift the sheet from your horse's head. Don't forget to refasten the snap to your horse's halter.

USING A
BLANKET ROLLER

A roller is a surcingle designed to hold a sheet or blanket in place. Rollers are made of leather, web, elastic, or a combination of materials. If a sheet or blanket fits properly and has hind leg straps, you won't need to use a roller. The sheet in these photos does not need one but is used for demonstration purposes. If you have a sheet without leg straps and it tends to shift to the left or right, a roller might provide enough stability to keep the blanket in place.

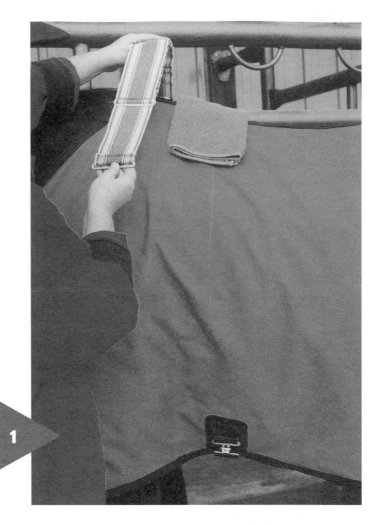

1 ▶ After the sheet is in place and all buckles are fastened, place a small hand towel or wither pad just behind the horse's withers. This padding will prevent the surcingle from creating pressure sores on the horse's back.

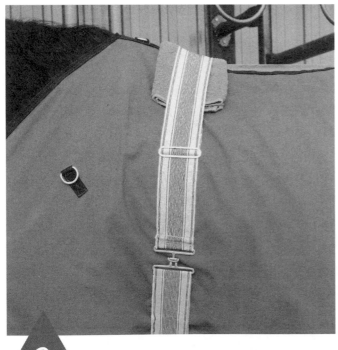

2 ▶ Place the surcingle on top of the pad and buckle it.

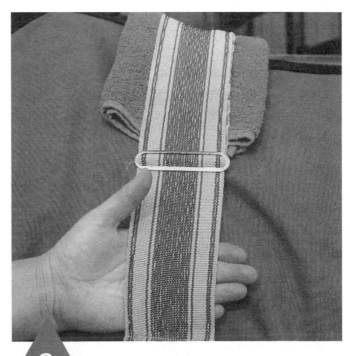

3 ▶ The surcingle should be adjusted so that you can still slip a hand easily underneath it, but not so loose that it won't do any good.

PUTTING ON A HOOD

The best place to put a hood on your horse is in the stall, because you won't have to deal with a halter.

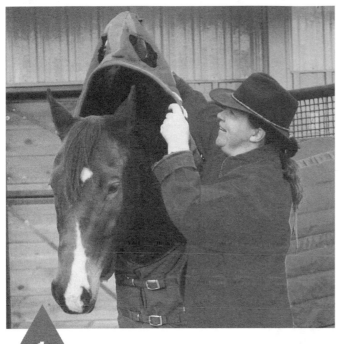

1 Unbuckle the hood and place one side on each side of the horse's neck behind his ears. Lift the hood up and bring it forward.

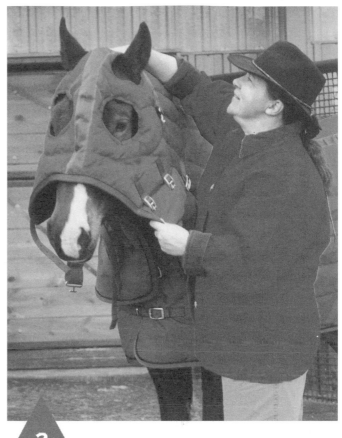

2 Lower it onto your horse's face, taking care not to bump his eyes as you position it.

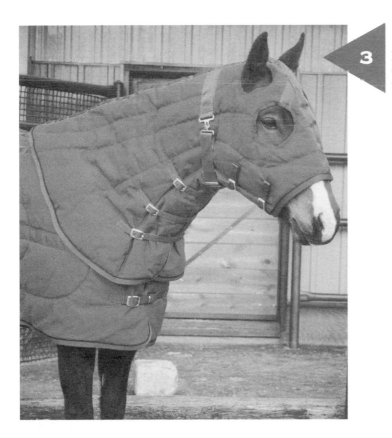

3 Adjust the straps so the hood fits well. Attach the hood to the blanket via the three straps that are customarily provided.

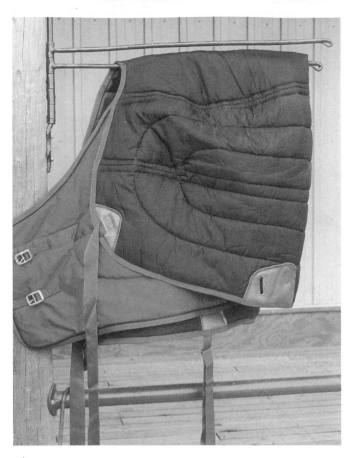

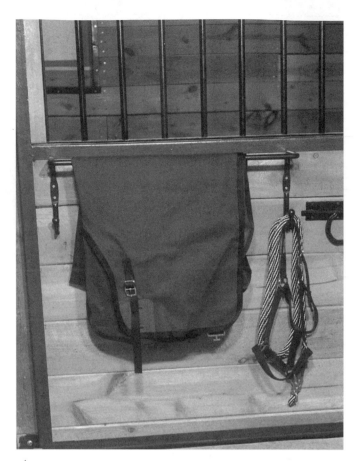

▲
HANG BLANKETS IN THE SUN

When you take a blanket off your horse so that you can work or ride him, hang it inside out on a blanket rack in the sun. The sunlight will freshen the inside of the blanket while the horse is being worked. The blanket will be ready to put on the horse after he has cooled down from the ride.

▲
HANDY BLANKET RACK

In the spring and fall, a warm blanket must often be changed to a lighter sheet during the heat of the day. It is handy for each stall to have a blanket bar to hold this "change of clothing."

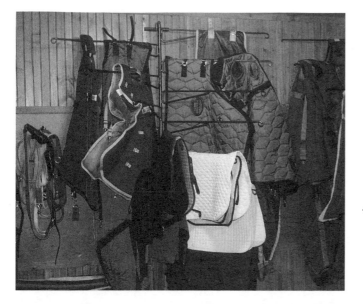

◀ STORE BLANKETS CLEAN

When a blanket is not in use, it should be washed and dried thoroughly. It can be stored on a blanket rack, such as this multipurpose horse and saddle blanket rack.

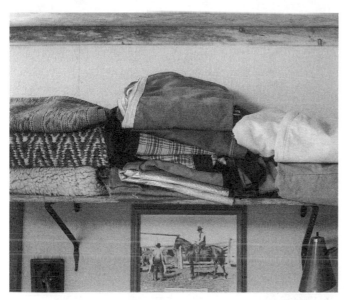

◀ STORING THIN SHEETS AND BLANKETS

Thin sheets and blankets can be folded and stored in a pile on a shelf. An alternative is to store them in a cupboard or in a trunk. The storage areas must be absolutely rodent-free, insectproof, and dry.

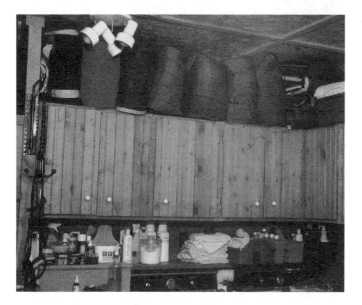

◀ STORING THICK BLANKETS

Thick, fluffy winter blankets should be rolled and stored in a way that won't compress them.

CLEANING HOOK-AND-LOOP CLOSURES

Hook-and-loop fasteners (known also under the tradename Velcro) are common on horse clothing and tack. If handled properly, they provide years of use.

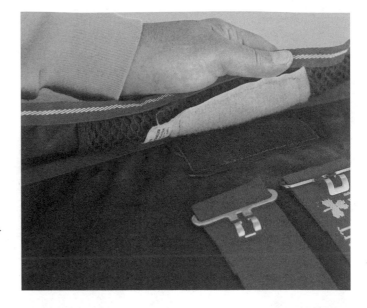

NOTE ▶

Before washing these items, fasten the hook-and-loop closures securely. Otherwise, the hook surface will invariably pick up a thick pad of horse hair and lint.

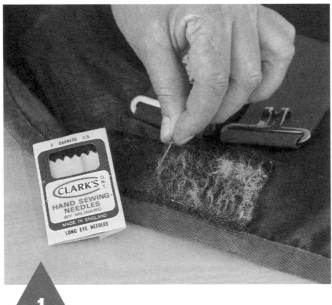

1 When this does happen, loosen the undesirable debris clogging the hooks by running a large darning needle between the rows of hooks. This loosens and lifts the hair pad.

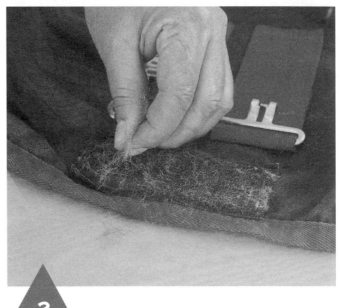

2 Much of the hair can then be lifted up with the fingers.

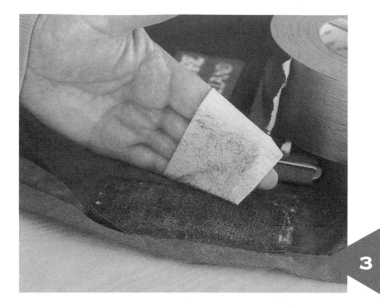

3 Loose hairs can be lifted out using strips of duct tape.

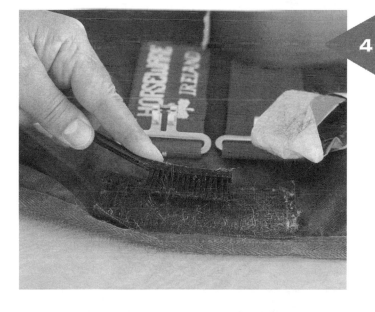

4 The final cleaning can be with a brush.

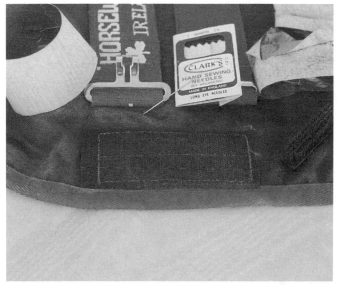

◀ THE FINISHED PRODUCT
Hook-and-loop closures work best when they have been cleaned. Store them with the closures fastened securely.

Appendix

PARTS OF THE HORSE

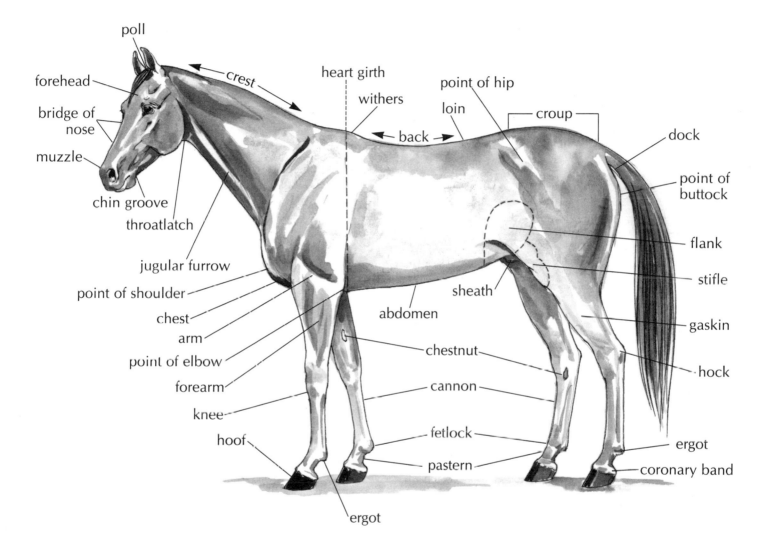

poll

forehead

crest

heart girth

point of hip

bridge of nose

withers

loin

croup

dock

muzzle

back

point of buttock

chin groove

throatlatch

flank

jugular furrow

sheath

stifle

point of shoulder

abdomen

gaskin

chest

chestnut

arm

hock

point of elbow

forearm

cannon

knee

fetlock

ergot

hoof

pastern

coronary band

ergot

Quick-Release Knot

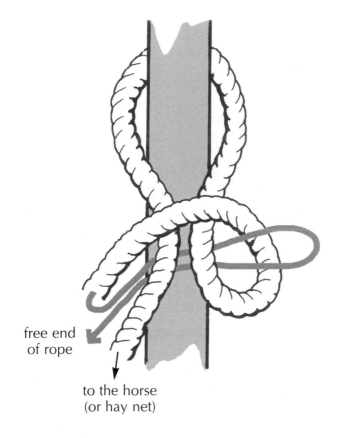

free end
of rope

to the horse
(or hay net)

free end
of rope

to the horse
(or hay net)

Wrap the rope around a post or object you are tying to. Make a loop with the free end on top. Double the free end and pass it though the loop.

When you pull the free end, it releases the knot quickly.

Recommended Reading

Haas, Jessie. *Safe Horse, Safe Rider: A Young Rider's Guide to Responsible Horsekeeping.* Pownal, VT: Storey Publishing, 1994.

Hayes, Karen, DVM. *Emergency! The Active Horseman's Book of Emergency Care.* Middletown, MD: Half Halt Press, 1995.

Hill, Cherry. *101 Arena Exercises: A Ringside Guide for Horse and Rider.* Pownal, VT: Storey Publishing, 1995.

———. *Becoming an Effective Rider: Developing Your Mind and Body for Balance and Unity.* Pownal, VT: Garden Way, 1991.

———. *The Formative Years: Raising and Training the Horse from Birth to Two Years.* Ossining, NY: Breakthrough, 1988.

———. *From the Center of the Ring: An Inside View of Horse Competitions.* Pownal, VT: Garden Way, 1988.

———. *Horse for Sale: How to Buy a Horse or Sell the One You Have.* New York, NY: Howell Book House, 1995.

———. *Horse Handling & Grooming: A Step-by-Step Photographic Guide to Mastering over 100 Horsekeeping Skills.* Pownal, VT: Storey Publishing, 1997.

———. *Horsekeeping on a Small Acreage: Facilities Design and Management.* Pownal, VT: Garden Way, 1990.

———. *Making Not Breaking: The First Year Under Saddle.* Ossining, NY: Breakthrough, 1992.

———. *Your Pony, Your Horse: A Kid's Guide to Care and Enjoyment.* Pownal, VT: Storey Publishing, 1995.

Hill, Cherry, and Richard Klimesh, CJF. *Maximum Hoof Power: How to Improve Your Horse's Performance through Proper Hoof Management.* New York, NY: Howell Book House, 1994.

Kellon, Eleanor, VMD. *Dr. Kellon's Guide to First Aid for Horses.* Ossining, NY: Breakthrough, 1990.

Lewis, Lon. *Feeding and Care of the Horse,* second edition. Baltimore, MD: Williams & Wilkins, 1995.

Lloyd, Sharon. *Clipping Horses and Ponies: A Complete Illustrated Manual.* Middletown, MD: Half Halt Press, 1995.

Stashak, Ted, DVM, and Cherry Hill. *Horseowner's Guide to Lameness.* Baltimore, MD: Williams & Wilkins, 1995.

Glossary

ABRASION. Scrape.

ASCARIDS. Roundworms.

ASPIRATE. Pull back slightly on syringe plunger to draw fluid back into chamber (checks whether needle has entered a blood vessel).

BLANCH. Temporarily squeeze the blood out of capillaries.

BOTS. *Gasterophilus*; Parasitic flies.

BOWED TENDON. Inflammation of the flexor tendon.

BRIDLE PATH. The 4" to 6" area between the forelock and the mane that is usually clipped.

CLINCHES. The folded-over ends of horseshoe nails on the outside of a shod horse's hooves.

CONJUNCTIVITIS. Inflammation of the conjunctiva of the eyes.

CONJUNCTIVA. The white membrane that lines the eyelid.

DERMATITIS. Inflammation of the dermal layer (outer layer) of the skin.

DIVERTICULUM. Blind pouch (a pocket or closed branch).

ELECTROLYTES. Minerals necessary for many body functions.

EXTENSOR TENDONS. Tendons located at the front of a limb.

FLEHMEN. A reaction to odd smells or tastes; horse curls upper lip upward.

FLEXOR TENDONS. Tendons located at the rear of a limb.

GALVAYNE'S GROOVE. V-shaped groove that appears at the gum line of the corner incisor at age of 10.

HEAT. The time in the mare's breeding cycle when she is "hot" or receptive to the stallion.

INTERDENTAL SPACE. A relatively toothless space between the premolars and the incisors.

INTRAMUSCULAR (IM). In the muscle.

INTRAVENOUS. In the vein.

INVERSION. A dangerous condition where a horse's respiration rate is higher than its pulse rate.

LACERATION. Cut.

LARVAE. Maggots.

NEOPRENE. Closed cell foam.

PARROT MOUTH. An overbite; the upper incisors hang over the lower incisors.

PINWORMS. *Oxyuris equi*; parasites.

PREMOLARS. The teeth that are located in front of the molars.

RHINOPNEUMONITIS. A respiratory illness.

SERUM. The watery portion of the blood that sometimes oozes through the skin.

SMEGMA. Accumulation of fatty secretions, dead skin cells, and dirt found in the male's sheath.

STRONGYLES. Bloodworms.

SUBCUTANEOUS. Under the skin.

SURCINGLE. The strap that encircles the heart girth.

TURGOR. Normal state of distention and resiliency of the skin.

Index

Page references in *italics* indicate illustrations.

OTHER STOREY TITLES YOU WILL ENJOY

101 Arena Exercises: A Ringside Guide for Horse & Rider, by Cherry Hill. A ringside exercise book for riders who want to improve their own and their horses' skills. Classic exercises and original patterns and drills presented in a unique "read and ride" format. 224 pages. Paperback. ISBN 0-88266-316-X.

Becoming an Effective Rider: Developing Your Mind and Body for Balance and Unity, by Cherry Hill. Teaches riders how to evaluate their own skills, plan a work session, get maximum use out of lesson time, set goals and achieve them, and protect themselves from injury. 192 pages. Paperback. ISBN 0-88266-688-6.

Fences for Pasture & Garden, by Gail Damerow. The complete guide to choosing, planning, and building today's best fences: wire, rail, electric, high-tension, temporary, woven, and snow. Also chapters on gates and trellises. 160 pages. Paperback. ISBN 0-88266-753-X.

The Horse Doctor Is In, by Brent Kelley, DVM. Kelley covers all aspects of horse health care, from fertility to fractures to foot care using real-life stories from his 30 years of experience as an equine vet. 320 pages. Paperback. ISBN 1-58017-460-4.

Horse Handling & Grooming: A Step-by-Step Photographic Guide, by Cherry Hill. This user-friendly guide to essential skills includes feeding, haltering, tying, grooming, clipping, bathing, braiding, and blanketing. The wealth of practical advice offered is thorough enough for beginners, yet useful for experienced riders improving or expanding their skills. 160 pages. Paperback. ISBN 0-88266-956-7.

Horsekeeping on a Small Acreage: Facilities Design and Management, by Cherry Hill. Horse trainer Cherry Hill describes the essentials for designing safe and functional facilities. 192 pages. Paperback. ISBN 0-88266-596-0.

Horse Sense: A Complete Guide to Horse Selection & Care, by John J. Mettler Jr., DVM. The basics on selecting, housing, fencing, and feeding a horse including information on immunizations, dental care, and breeding. 160 pages. Paperback. ISBN 0-88266-545-6.

Keeping Livestock Healthy: A Veterinary Guide to Horses, Cattle, Pigs, Goats & Sheep, by N. Bruce Haynes, DVM. Provides in-depth tips on how to prevent disease through good nutrition, proper housing, and the appropriate care. Includes an overview of the dozens of diseases and the latest information on technologies livestock owners need to know. 352 pages. Paperback. ISBN 0-88266-884-6.

Safe Horse, Safe Rider: A Young Rider's Guide to Responsible Horsekeeping, by Jessie Haas. Beginning with understanding the horse and ending with competitions, every chapter includes encouraging ideas for a good relationship. Chapters on horse body language, safe pastures and stables, catching, leading and tying, grooming safety, and riding out. 160 pages. Paperback. ISBN 0-88266-700-9.

Your Horse: A Step-by-Step Guide to Horse Ownership, by Judy Chapple. Highly readable for all ages and packed with practical information on buying, housing, feeding, training, riding, and handling medical problems. 144 pages. Paperback. ISBN 0-88266-353-4.

Your Pony, Your Horse: A Kid's Guide to Care and Enjoyment, by Cherry Hill. Part of our friendly and encouraging children's animal reference series, featuring information on selection, housing, feeding, health, behavior, and showing in mature yet easy-to-understand language. 160 pages. Paperback. ISBN 0-88266-908-7.

The Illustrated Guide to Horse Tack for the English Rider, by Susan McBane. With this book in hand, buyers of horse-related clothing and equipment will be well prepared to make informed purchasing decisions the first time around. 198 pages. Hardcover. ISBN 0-88266-879-X.

Western Riding, by Charlene Strickland. This book goes beyond the traditional teachings to be the rider's one-stop Western riding guide. From a review of breeds and basic handling to enthusiastic instructions on various Western riding disciplines to tips from professional coaches, this book is much more than how to ride, rope, and race. 272 pages. Hardcover. ISBN 0-88266-890-0.

These and other books from Storey Publishing are available wherever quality books are sold or by call 1-800-441-5700.
Visit us at www.storey.com.